Property of George, Trammell & Battle

Please return

PRIORITIES IN MULTIPLE TRAUMA

reprinted from

TOPICS IN EMERGENCY MEDICINE

edited by
Harvey W. Meislin, M.D.

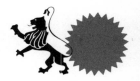

AN ASPEN PUBLICATION®
Aspen Systems Corporation
Germantown, Maryland
London, England
1980

Library of Congress Cataloging in Publication Data
Main entry under title:

Priorities in multiple trauma.

1. Wounds and injuries. 2. Emergency medicine.
3. Traumatology. I. Meislin, Harvey W. II. Topics
in emergency medicine. [DNLM: 1. Disaster planning.
2. Wounds and injuries. W0700 P958 1979a]
RD93.P74 1980   617'.2   80-11266
ISBN 0-89443-287-7

Copyright © 1980 by Aspen Systems Corporation

Library of Congress Catalog Card Number: 80-11266
ISBN: 0-89443-287-7

Printed in the United States of America

1 2 3 4 5

Contents

PRIORITIES IN MULTIPLE TRAUMA

Topics in Emergency Medicine
Editorial Board

Barry H. Rumack, M.D.
Director
Rocky Mountain Poison Center
Denver, Colorado

Mary Beth Skelton, R.N.
Director of Paramedic Training
School of Medicine
Tulane University
New Orleans, Louisiana

Ronald O. Stewart, M.D.
Medical Director
Emergency Department
Presbyterian University Hospital
Pittsburgh, Pennsylvania

Wayne R. Tanner, M.S.W., A.C.S.W.
Weber State College
Department of Sociology,
    Anthropology and Social Work
Ogden, Utah

William L. Teufel, M.D.
Director
Emergency Service
San Francisco General Hospital
Assistant Clinical Professor of Surgery
University of California
San Francisco, California

Gail Walraven
EMS Consultant
Long Beach, California

Susan L. Weed
Executive Director
American Trauma Society
Chicago, Illinois

Issue Editor/Author:

Harvey W. Meislin, M.D.
Associate Director
Emergency Medicine Center
UCLA Hospital and Clinics
Los Angeles, California

Authors:

Paul S. Auerbach, M.D.
Junior Resident
UCLA Center for the Health Sciences
Department of Emergency Medicine
Los Angeles, California

Frank J. Baker, II, M.D.
Associate Professor and Director
Department of Emergency Medicine
The University of Chicago Hospitals and Clinics
Chicago, Illinois

Cathy L. Box, R.N., M.I.C.N.
Clinical Nurse Instructor
Department of Emergency Health Services
Truman Medical Center
School of Medicine
University of Missouri Kansas City
Kansas City, Missouri

Robert S. Brown, M.D.
Division Head
Division of Trauma Surgery
Henry Ford Hospital
Detroit, Michigan

Jill E. Furgurson, M.D.
Emergency Medicine Resident
Emergency Medicine Center
UCLA Hospital and Clinics
Los Angeles, California

Martin S. Kohn, M.D.
Department of Emergency Medicine
Good Samaritan Hospital
San Jose, California

Larry N. Marcum, B.S., E.M.T.-P.
Director
San Juan Regional Medical Center
Emergency Medical Services
Farmington, New Mexico

Richard M. Nowak, M.D.
Senior Staff Physician
Division of Emergency Medicine
Henry Ford Hospital
Detroit, Michigan

James R. Roberts, M.D.
Assistant Professor in Emergency Medicine
The Medical College of Pennsylvania
Philadelphia, Pennsylvania

Robert J. Rothstein, M.D.
Assistant Professor and Associate Director
Department of Emergency Medicine
The University of Chicago Hospitals and Clinics
Chicago, Illinois

George Sternbach, M.D.
Assistant Medical Director
Emergency Services
Stanford University Medical Center
Stanford, California

Joe G. Talbert, M.D.
Senior Staff Physician
Division of Trauma Surgery
Henry Ford Hospital
Detroit, Michigan

Michael C. Tomlanovich, M.D.
Director
Residency Program
Division of Emergency Medicine
Henry Ford Hospital
Detroit, Michigan

Joseph F. Waeckerle, M.D.
Assistant Professor and Vice Chairman
Department of Emergency Health Services
Truman Medical Center
School of Medicine
University of Missouri Kansas City
Kansas City, Missouri

From the editors . . .

Topics in Emergency Medicine (TEM) was conceived of and designed to provide a unique journal for all emergency medicine clinicians (physicians, nurses and paramedics) functioning as individuals committed to quality care. It is designed to provide a vehicle for advanced and continuing education, research findings with practical applications and other meaningful topics of interest in the field.

Emergency medicine, as both a science and an art, represents a dynamic force in holistic health care which utilizes clinicians operating as a single goal-directed unit striving toward the achievement of the optimum in emergency medical care. It is in the belief that all emergency medicine clinicians function as peers that this journal has its roots. This intradisciplinary approach is geared toward continuity and coordination of total services for individuals, families and their communities in a fashion not previously addressed in existing professional journals.

Predicated upon the philosophy of TEM, the editors hope to establish strong communication, efficient functional linkages and mutual respect among the various disciplines. Concomitant with this developmental growth is the process of accurately assessing emergency needs, formulating a definitive diagnosis, developing a strong plan of management, and implementing and evaluating intervention.

The editors of TEM believe that intervention for the critically ill and injured does not originate in the emergency department; rather it originates at the site of the onset of illness or injury. Thus TEM will place emphasis within each issue on the critical aspect of prehospital intervention.

In addition to prehospital care, this journal advocates the principle of dynamic and comprehensive management. Within this framework, management embraces prehospital intervention, emergency department treatment, an expanded concept of critical care and rehabilitative follow-through.

Unlike current standards for emergency medicine, the standards on which TEM is founded hold that the responsibility of emergency medicine clinicians extends beyond the emergency department. Realization of this goal would witness the integration and/or coordination within and among each of the intervention phases of the patient care continuum.

Unless each phase of the patient care continuum can be fulfilled the holistic concept is incomplete.

Service delivery is only as effective as its educational supporting foundation. The importance of ongoing education in the field of emergency medicine incorporates the broad scope of physical, psychological and sociological dimensions of treatment. Because these three aspects of human existence are interrelated and interdependent, each must be considered within the context of holistic care.

TEM is pleased to introduce this journal as a forum for innovative concepts related to quality emergency medical care and its management.

—Carmen Germaine Warner, R.N., P.H.N.
—Marc J. Bayer, M.D.
—Knut F. Eie, Paramedic
Editors

Foreword

Trauma is the number one killer in the under-40-age group. How can we in medicine alter this extremely high phenomenon of morbidity and mortality? Studies have shown that the initial evaluation, resuscitation and stabilization may determine whether trauma victims survive. It is not the surgeons, it is not the subspecialists; it is the clinicians involved in emergency medicine who make the difference in these extreme situations. Emergency medicine physicians, nurses and paramedics all play a role in the team effort to salvage life and limb. The unique biology of emergency medicine demands that with a minimal amount of input, aggressive and appropriate stabilization and resuscitative measures be taken in the setting of the multiply traumatized victim. The emergency physician, as team leader, can organize all these efforts and mobilize the appropriate specialists which will lead to survival, if survival can be obtained.

This issue of *Topics in Emergency Medicine* is unique. It deals with a subject common to all emergency medicine clinicians. But its uniqueness lies in the articles themselves. All articles are written by on-line, first-hand clinicians who day in and day out deal with priorities in multiple trauma. Most of the authors have done their postdoctoral training in emergency medicine. Who is more appropriate than these emergency physicians, nurses and paramedics to discuss such topics as those appearing in this issue?

Although a journal can divide priorities in multiple trauma into several articles, in reality, the approach to multiple trauma is a continuum. It is the cyclic examination, evaluation and resuscitation that must occur over and over again until it is evident that a life or limb threat no longer exists. This evaluation takes place at all levels of sophistication, be it in the field, in the emergency department or in the operating suite. The authors have presented an excellent, succinct and current approach to the priorities of multiple trauma.

I would like to thank my colleagues who have authored the articles for sharing their expertise and talents in the type of journal that is very appropriate to emergency medicine—a journal that is topic oriented, to the point and current. I believe TEM will continue forth in the excellent manner demonstrated by the authors in this first issue.

—Harvey W. Meislin, M.D.
Issue Editor

Priorities in Multiple Systems Injuries

Larry N. Marcum, B.S., E.M.T.-P.
Director
San Juan Regional Medical Center
Emergency Medical Services
Farmington, New Mexico

Cathy L. Box, R.N., M.I.C.N.
Clinical Nurse Instructor
Department of Emergency Health Services
Truman Medical Center

Joseph F. Waeckerle, M.D.
Assistant Professor and Vice Chairman
Department of Emergency Health Services
Truman Medical Center
School of Medicine
University of Missouri Kansas City
Kansas City, Missouri

MORBIDITY AND MORTALITY associated with trauma are devastating, particularly since most deaths occur under the age of 40 years. Further compounding the tragedy is the fact that many deaths can be prevented if certain conditions are treated quickly and effectively. The priorities are to insure: (1) a patent airway, (2) adequate respiratory function, (3) adequate cardiovascular function, and (4) appropriate spinal immobilization. Death or further sequelae from injury most often result from lack of attention to these priorities. Emphasis must therefore be placed on a rapid initial survey of these functions. Only after essential systems are evaluated may a more detailed examination to provide additional treatment be indicated. The management priorities for trauma center around organ systems that best reflect hypoxia and inadequate tissue perfusion, the respiratory, cardiovascular and central nervous systems (CNSs).

2

PATHOPHYSIOLOGY

Quick assessment and intervention are more easily accomplished if emergency medicine clinicians understand the basic pathophysiology of acute trauma. Whenever the body suffers acute trauma, the sympathetic nervous system attempts to compensate. The resultant release of the endogenous catecholamines, epinephrine and norepinephrine, causes an increase in heart rate and stroke volume, and a selective vasoconstriction of the least essential vascular beds. Initially, this maintains adequate blood flow to vital organs. However, prolonged vasoconstriction forces inadequately perfused vascular beds to undergo anaerobic metabolism, which produces a lactic acidosis and is the reason for many of the sequelae of shock.

Although catecholamines also have an effect on the respiratory system, the main stimuli of respiration are hypoxia and/or hypercarbia. With an increase in carbon dioxide, the respiratory rate increases as the body tries to "blow-off" the excess carbon dioxide to correct the pH. In the face of acute trauma, the increased respiratory rate is usually not sufficient to compensate for the decreased tidal volume. The result is a serious ventilation/perfusion defect, which only compounds the overall problem of tissue hypoxia. The ventilation/perfusion mismatch results in less oxygen intake and more carbon dioxide retention. The hypoxemia further propagates the anaerobic cycle, and the hypercarbia increases the respiratory component of acidemia. Both also affect the respiratory center in the brain.

In conditions leading to oxygen deprivation, cerebral ischemia results. With an increase in carbon dioxide levels, vasodilatation of the cerebral vessels occurs. Such vasodilatation in the presence of intracerebral hemorrhage may increase the expanding hematoma, thereby eventually causing brain stem herniation, further compromising the cardiorespiratory functions. In the spinal cord, this vasodilatation contributes to the swelling associated with cord contusions, which can result in either partial or total neurological dysfunction below the site of injury.

Figures 1 and 2 depict the basic chain reactions that occur in acute respiratory and cardiovascular failure. It is important to emphasize that these reactions occur to some extent in almost every acute emergency.

RESPIRATORY SYSTEM

Securing a patent airway is the first priority of treatment in any patient who exhibits signs of actual or impending respiratory distress. The airway should be checked for vomitus, blood, teeth, tongue or foreign body obstruction; furthermore, noisy breathing, inspiratory stridor, tracheal tugging or accessory muscle use may indicate an obstruction. The location of the trachea should be noted and examined for evidence of local trauma. After assuring that the airway is patent, the respiratory rate must be checked. Concern should be aroused when the rate is less than eight or more than 25 times per minute. A rate of less than eight may not provide an adequate minute volume, especially if the tidal volume is also below normal; such a

FIGURE 1. PATHOPHYSIOLOGY IN ACUTE RESPIRATORY FAILURE

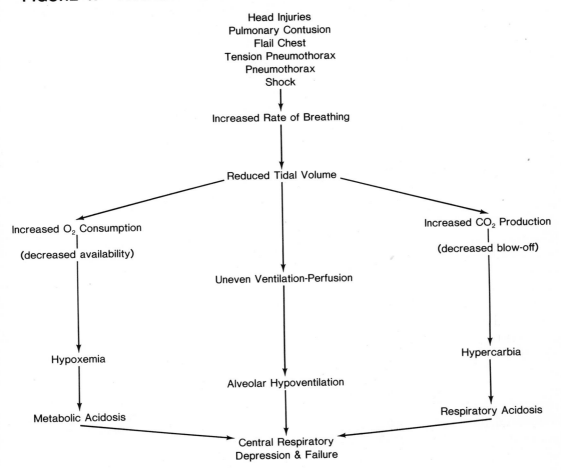

patient needs ventilatory assistance with oxygen. When in doubt concerning the adequacy of respiration, assist the patient. A rate of more than 25 per minute may be suggestive of acidosis and/or hypoxia.

The rhythm of the respiratory effort must be evaluated. An irregular pattern is serious, particularly Cheyne-Stoke's respirations and central neurogenic hyperventilation, which are most often associated with severe head injuries. Cheyne-Stoke's

respirations are characterized by slow and shallow breathing that gets progressively faster and deeper, then slower and shallow again, followed by a period of near or total apnea. The pattern then repeats itself. Central neurogenic hyperventilation is characterized by sustained rapid, deep breathing. Ataxic or agonal respiratory effort has no pattern and is a sign of terminal injury or illness. The final step in evaluation is to assess breath sounds bilat-

4

FIGURE 2.   PATHOPHYSIOLOGY IN CARDIOVASCULAR FAILURE

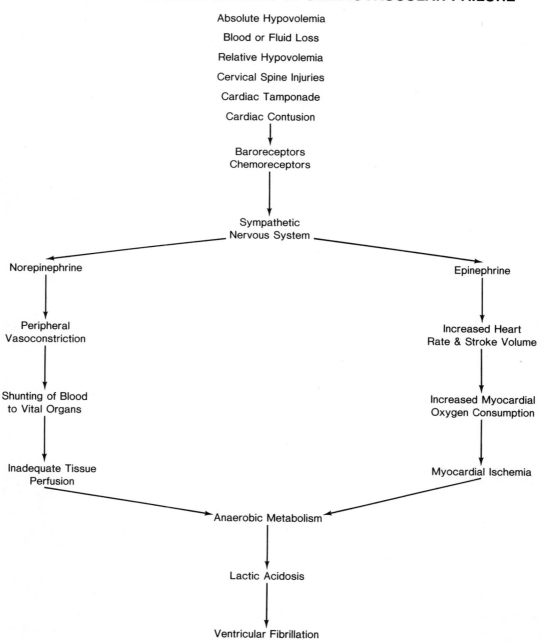

erally. The patient should have equal breath sounds in all lung fields. Diminished or absent sounds in the lower lobes indicates hypoventilation. Diminished or absent sounds on one side may indicate pneumothorax, which can be quickly lethal.

Treatment of respiratory distress should be begun under the premise that a cervical spine injury may be present, particularly with coma or obvious head trauma. The specific treatment used depends on: (1) the patient's condition, (2) the skills of the rescuer, and (3) the availability of equipment. Effective treatment may be as simple as opening the airway, turning the patient on the side to provide for drainage of secretions or suctioning. If the patient is breathing spontaneously, assistance may be provided by insertion of an oropharyngeal or nasopharyngeal airway. With absent or severe compromise of respiration, ventilation may be maintained by use of the bag-valve-mask with oxygen or by oxygen-powered breathing devices. In more severe cases, the passage of an esophageal airway or intubation by oral or nasal routes, in conjunction with bag-valves or oxygen-powered breathing devices may be needed. The final consideration would be cricothyrotomy or emergency tracheostomy in certain selective cases.

The importance of oxygen in assisted ventilation cannot be overemphasized; its deprivation results in anaerobic metabolism and lactic acidosis. Oxygen can reverse the process of local tissue hypoxia. With acidosis, oxygen disassociation with hemoglobin and oxygen delivery to the tissues are enhanced; however, there is also a lesser oxygen saturation of hemoglobin at any given PaO_2. Increasing the PaO_2 and, therefore, the oxygen saturation of hemoglobin insures a more adequate delivery of oxygen to the tissues.

CARDIOVASCULAR SYSTEM

The release of catecholamines is responsible for many cardiovascular signs and symptoms. Epinephrine and norepinephrine cause the skin to become pale, cool and diaphoretic, the pupils to dilate, and the systolic blood pressure to be maintained at a relatively normal level in a hypovolemic patient. For this reason, a normal blood pressure does not rule out serious injuries. In the adult, blood pressure may be normal, even after a liter of fluid has been lost by compensating with an increased heart rate and shunting intravascular volume. When palpating the pulse, rate and quality as well as alternating strengths and weaknesses should be noted. Pulsus alternans, fluctuation in pulse strength, may indicate cardiac tamponade, tension pneumothorax or acute hypovolemia.

Hypovolemia and hypotension must be treated aggressively. Initial treatment should be to control external hemorrhage. For patients presenting with the signs and symptoms of shock or who have sustained multiple trauma, one or more large-bore intravenous lines should be started using balanced salt solutions. The rapid infusion of solutions in head injury patients is contraindicated unless the patient is in shock. In such cases, the treatment of shock takes priority over the head injury since shock is very unlikely with an

6

isolated head injury and indicates other bleeding injuries.

Antishock trousers are an effective adjunct in the treatment of hypovolemia and shock, especially with intravenous fluid administration. Shock trousers transfer approximately 750 to 1000 ml of blood from the lower extremities and abdomen to the central circulation. They were, at one time, thought to be contraindicated in patients with head and chest injuries because the increased blood to these areas was thought to promote bleeding. This has not been confirmed when the patient is hypovolemic. Another relative contraindication was trauma with concomitant respiratory embarrassment. In these cases, the benefits derived from the trousers exceed the decrease in respiratory function if the patient is closely observed and respiratory distress is aggressively treated.

NEUROLOGICAL SYSTEM

Changes in the level of consciousness and aberrations of sensorium are often the first clues to the patient's condition. In acute multiple systems trauma, hypoxia and shock as well as head injury, must be considered as the cause of these changes. Level of consciousness should be described in objective terms, for example, "alert," "responsive to verbal and/or painful stimuli" or "unresponsive to verbal and/or painful stimuli." Stimulation may cause the patient to assume a decorticate or decerebrate posture, which are ominous signs. In evaluating consciousness, the pupils are important. The pupillary response is governed by the third cranial nerve, and the pupils respond to blood

oxygen concentrations and light. An abnormal response or no response in a patient without a history of eye pathology usually indicates damage from trauma or hypoperfusion-hypoxia of the central nervous system.

Injuries to the spinal column and cord commonly accompany head injuries and should receive high priority to prevent complications. Many injuries can be averted, limited or possibly reversed with proper care before arrival at the hospital. The following signs or symptoms suggest spinal cord injury: (1) paralysis or weakness of the extremities, particularly if bilateral; (2) paresthesia or tingling sensations in the trunk or any of the extremities; (3) loss of bladder and bowel function; (4) pain or deformity in any region of the spine; (5) stiffness or pain in the neck referred to the shoulder or arms; (6) any trauma victim who is unable to respond appropriately; (7) any trauma patient whose respiratory effort resembles abdominal breathing; and (8) shock of unknown origin, especially when associated with vasodilatation and warm, dry skin.

Since the spinal cord is approximately one-half inch in diameter and the spinal canal only five-eighths inch in diameter, there is not much room for swelling, which is mainly responsible for morbidity in patients. The bony injuries to the spine are not as important as how they affect the neuroanatomy within the canal. It is imperative that the head, neck and spine of the patient with multiple injuries be immobilized by spine boards, firm cervical collars and sandbags to protect against spinal cord damage. The use of each is indicated by numerous findings, most important of which is the position of the patient. The head should be in neutral position, neither flexed nor extended, during the extrication and immobilization. If the head must be moved prior to immobilization, this is best accomplished by applying gentle, in-line axial traction. The patient should not be moved until secured on a spine board unless the patient is in clear danger by remaining in the immediate environment of the trauma scene.

SUMMARY

It is essential to approach the patient with multiple trauma with a plan, which insures an adequate examination to rule out life-threatening injuries. Clinicians who are well schooled, disciplined and efficient in carrying out such a plan can increase patient survival. This was demonstrated during the Vietnam war when battlefield mortality was decreased to approximately 1% through on-site treatment and efficient management at the base hospital. An examination for less essential injuries may be carried out at the scene, in transit or upon arrival at the emergency department, contingent upon the time and conditions surrounding the patient's care.

Management of the patient with multiple systems injury presents an unparalleled challenge to the emergency medical clinician. To give the best possible emergency treatment, assuring proper care of airway, ventilation, circulation and spinal cord must be the priorities.

SUGGESTED READINGS

Ballinger V, Rutherford R, Zuidema G: *The Management of Trauma.* Philadelphia, WB Saunders Co, 1973, pp 144–218.

Caldwell RB: Epidural Hematoma—a true emergency. *JACEP* 4:49–50, January–February 1975.

Carey LC: Shock: differential diagnosis and immediate treatment. *Hosp Med* 68–93, May 1975.

Dillman PA: The biophysical response to shock trousers. *J Emer Nurs* 3(6): 21–25, November–December 1977.

Dragosa T: Brainstem damage associated with cerebral injury. *Emergency Nurs* 2:9–14, September–October 1976.

Goldman A: Respiratory distress: diagnosis and emergency management. *Emergency Med Servs* September–October 1977.

Hitchcock ER: Treatment of head injuries. *Nurs Times* 70:1193–1195, August 1974.

Jahre JA, Grace WJ, Greenbaum DM et al: Medical approach to the hypotensive patient and the patient in shock. *Heart Lung* 4(4):577–586, July–August 1975.

Krieger AJ: Getting down to cases—the head. *Emergency Med* February 1976.

Lilja GP, Batalden DJ, Adams BE, et al: Value of the counterpressure suit (MAST) in pre-hospital care. *Minn Med* 58:540–543, July 1975.

Miller RH, Cantrell FR: *Textbook of Basic Emergency Medicine.* St Louis, CV Mosby Co, 1975.

Ransom K, McSwain N: Respiratory function following application of MAST trousers. *JACEP* 7(8):297–299, August 1978.

Romano T: Initial evaluation of the multiple injury patient. *Emergency Med Servs* (4):24–30, July–August 1976.

Sproul C, Mulhaney PJ: *Emergency Care: Asssessment and Intervention.* St Louis, CV Mosby Co, 1974.

Swift N: Head injury. *Nurs Magazine* 4(9):26–33, September 1974.

US Department of Transportation, National Highway Safety Administration: *Emergency Care in the Field, A Manual for Paramedics.* Washington DC, Government Printing Office.

Weiss M: Axioms on the management of head injury. *Hosp Med* 94–110, May 1975.

Wilkins EW, Jr.: *Textbook of Emergency Medicine.* Baltimore, Williams and Wilkins Co, 1978.

Airway Problems in the Trauma Victim

Jill E. Furgurson, M.D.
Emergency Medicine Resident

Harvey W. Meislin, M.D.
Associate Director
Emergency Medicine Center
UCLA Hospital and Clinics
Los Angeles, California

ACCIDENTS ARE the leading causes of death in people under 40 years of age. Since respiratory problems and hemorrhage are the main acute causes of trauma-associated death, emergency medicine clinicians must insure adequate airway management in the trauma victim. The physician often has no prior knowledge of the patient's medical history with respect to lung disease or other cardiopulmonary ailments. In addition, the trauma patient may be barely conscious due to cerebral anoxia, hypovolemia, intoxication or cerebral injury. Such a patient therefore is a prime candidate for potential aspiration and upper airway obstruction. Airway embarrassment may be secondary to blunt or penetrating trauma to the neck, face or rib cage. Vascular injuries, impaled or foreign bodies may add additional complications.

Simple maneuvers to open an obstructed airway may be lifesaving, since it is often not the trauma itself that causes death, but the associated respiratory

10 embarrassment. The Vietnam experience revealed respiratory failure to be the most common cause of death in wounded soldiers who were transported to the hospital.[1]

INITIAL ASSESSMENT AND TREATMENT

A quick examination often reveals whether the patient is breathing adequately. To evaluate airway patency, clinicians must look, feel and listen. First, look to see if the patient's chest is rising and falling with respiration. Marked activity of the accessory muscles of respiration in the neck, supraclavicular and intercostal areas indicate possible airway compromise. Feel for movement of air through the patient's nose and mouth. If the patient is making respiratory efforts, and air flow cannot be ascertained, the airway is obstructed.

Listen to the patient. When airway obstruction is complete, air flow is not heard. Partial airway obstruction produces considerable noise of various frequency and intensity. The sounds can indicate the degree and location of obstruction. Upper airway obstruction is characterized by inspiratory stridor, whereas lower airway obstruction usually produces expiratory wheezes or stridor. Snoring is probably the best example of upper airway obstruction, caused by partial pharyngeal obstruction. Partial obstruction of the bronchi produces the wheezing effect so characteristic of asthma. Both inspiratory and expiratory stridor and/or wheezes may occur in upper and lower airway obstruction. Auscultation of the chest and signs of blunt or penetrating trauma may result in a diagnosis of pneumothorax, rib fractures or flail

chest. These conditions are discussed in the management of chest injury.

Most trauma victims hyperventilate at a rate often one and a half to two times normal rate, or 18 to 24 times a minute. This is due to a combination of factors including the stress of trauma. A patient who is not ventilating at a greater than normal respiratory rate should be suspected of having ventilatory problems in the airway, diaphragm, lungs, chest wall and/or the central nervous system (CNS).

Before using any airway adjuncts in a patient with signs of airway obstruction, simple techniques may relieve possible upper airway obstruction from the tongue and soft tissues of the hypopharynx. The three techniques (see Figure 1) utilized are:

1. *The Neck Lift.* With the patient lying supine, place one hand under the neck and the other on the forehead. Lift and extend the neck while tilting the head backwards by pressure on the forehead.

2. *The Chin Lift.* Place the fingers of one hand under the lower jaw at the chin and lift to bring the chin forward. Press on the forehead with the other hand to tilt the head backwards. The chin lift is the most adequate and consistent means of relieving airway obstruction.

3. *The Jaw Thrust.* Grab the angles of the mandible with both hands, one on each side, lifting and displacing it forward and thus opening the airway.[2]

If these maneuvers do not help, the oropharynx should be inspected to rule out possible obstructions such as loose teeth, dentures, vomitus, blood clots or mucus. Cleansing the airway when there is

FIGURE 1. TECHNIQUES FOR OPENING AN OBSTRUCTED AIRWAY

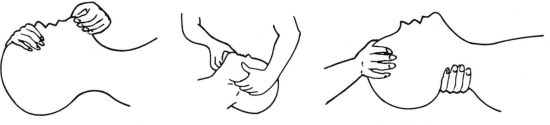

The Chin Lift   The Jaw Thrust   The Neck Lift

no cervical spine injury is accomplished by turning the patient's head to the side while pulling the jaw forward and extending the neck. All secretions should be suctioned or manually removed until the mouth and posterior pharynx are clean upon inspection. If there is any evidence or suspicion of neck injury or if cervical spine injury may result, the patient should be log-rolled in one continuous motion to the side to cleanse the airway. The procedures for assessing and cleansing the patient's airway and positioning the patient for the airway patency can be used to alleviate most causes of obstruction, whether or not the patient is in the hospital.

Once the maneuvers have been performed and if the patient is not alert, an oral or nasal airway should be inserted to prevent soft-tissue airway obstruction. In the semi-alert patient, the nasal airway tends to be better tolerated. A good rule of thumb for removal of an oral airway is when the patient gags or spits it out.

MAXILLOFACIAL TRAUMA

Automobile accidents are the most frequent cause of facial injuries. Investigations have shown 75% of all deaths and injuries from auto deceleration accidents include maxillofacial injuries caused by the head striking an unyielding object.[3] Other causes of facial injuries include fist fights, dog bites, epileptic seizures, bicycle and motorcycle accidents, falls and various athletic and recreational activities.

Facial fractures can be diagnosed by inspection, palpation and x-ray examination. Inspection begins with evaluation of the patient as a whole, assessment of pain and gross anatomical comparison of the two sides of the face. Localized ecchymosis or swelling should arouse suspicion of underlying fracture. Asymmetry secondary to trauma is usually obvious and an important observation. Bilateral palpation should be performed systematically to avoid missing subtle deformities. Beginning superiorly, the following should be noted: (1) supraorbital, lateral and inferior orbital rims; (2) malar eminences; (3) zygomatic arches; (4) nasal bones; (5) maxilla; and (6) mandible.[4] X-ray examination usually confirms the diagnosis. The single most informative x-ray view of the facial bone is the Waters' view. Other views should be obtained depending upon the patient's clinical presentation.

Priorities of stabilization in patients with

12 extensive facial trauma should always be the same. In order of importance, the following should be assessed and treated: airway, hemorrhage, assessment of associated injury, then local injury. The principal cause of death from facial injuries is obstruction of the upper airway. If a patient with facial trauma presents with signs of airway obstruction, the maneuvers previously described should be attempted first. If they fail, remove any blood clots or foreign bodies from the airway. The patient's dentures may be found driven back into the throat. A fractured mandibular arch may collapse and allow the base of the tongue to obstruct the entrance to the larynx. In such cases, a large towel clip or suture may be passed through the anterior tongue and traction used to bring both the tongue and the mandibular arch forward. If this does not produce an immediate gratifying in-rush of air, the examiner should check the position of the maxilla and soft palate. These structures may be impacted downward and backward to obstruct the oropharynx. If this is the problem, the fingers should be passed up behind the free edge of the displaced soft palate attempting to forcefully elevate the obstructed bones and soft tissues.

The Heimlich maneuver may relieve upper airway obstruction by foreign bodies lodged in the trachea. With the patient in the supine position, two force compressions are delivered to the epigastrium in a cephalad direction. The examiner should then check the oropharynx to extract any foreign body.

Deep lacerations of the face involving the nose, cheeks or palate, and compound fractures of the jaws bleed profusely. Blood clots may obstruct the airway.

Hemorrhage into the lungs may literally "drown" the patient. When airway obstruction is secondary to hemorrhage, the initial management should include: (1) manual extraction of the blood clots, (2) attempts to control bleeding, (3) placement of the patient in a prone position with the head to the side (unless cervical spine injury is suspected) and (4) suction through nasotracheal tube.[5] If the patient's clinical status allows, cross table x-rays of the neck should be taken immediately to rule out cervical spine injury.

If these initial measures do not quickly relieve the obstruction and cervical spine injury is not suspected, endotracheal intubation should be attempted. If efforts at intubation prove unsuccessful, cricothyroidotomy or transtracheal ventilation is performed. One of these procedures should be performed immediately in patients with proven or possible cervical spine injury who are apneic or in severe respiratory distress. Careful consideration must be given to patients with severe maxillofacial trauma even if they present with no symptoms or signs of airway compromise. Respiratory problems may develop hours later when hemorrhage into soft tissues and progressive edema produce airway occlusion. Delayed, occult hemorrhage may drown the obtunded patient if the airway is not protected. Anticipation of problems and frequent reevaluation of the airway status is of utmost importance.

LARYNGOTRACHEAL TRAUMA

Mid-airway obstruction may be produced by blunt or penetrating trauma to the laryngotracheal skeleton. Penetrating trauma to the neck is usually produced by gunshots and/or stab wounds of the neck, is usually apparent on physical examination and certainly calls attention to possible upper airway injury.

The most common cause of blunt injury to the neck is direct impact during an automobile collision. Other causes include falls or direct blows to the laryngotracheal areas, usually sustained in sports or pugilistic activities. The true incidence of laryngotracheal trauma is unknown; however, it is apparently increasing because of high speed automobile travel and civilian violence.[6] Injury to the trachea may immediately threaten the patient's life as well as contribute to long-term disability. Prompt recognition of such an injury, which is not always clinically obvious, is of utmost importance. Not uncommonly, extensive destruction of the laryngotracheal complex from blunt injury may clinically appear to be minor and therefore a high index of suspicion is required to assess the true situation. Fortunately, severe injuries to the laryngotracheal skeleton occur infrequently because the airway is protected by neck muscles, sternum, vertebral column and mandible. The mobility, elasticity and resiliency of the laryngotrachea and its cartilaginous support minimize injury.

Cervical spine and neck injuries often occur with rear-end auto collisions, in which the patient's neck is forced into sudden hyperextension. As a rule, injury to the trachea or larynx is not produced in this fashion. An interesting exception to this was recently treated at the UCLA Emergency Medicine Center. A patient, smoking marihuana, was in the midst of a Valsalva maneuver at the time his vehicle was involved in a rear-end collision. The patient sustained a tracheal tear due to the combination of the collision and the Valsalva, but he recovered uneventfully.

Head-on or frontal auto collision results in more frequent laryngotracheal morbidity. In these instances, the driver, usually not wearing a seatbelt, is thrown forward until the upper abdomen and lower chest strike the lower portion of the steering wheel. At this point, the head begins to flex forward. The trachea and larynx are usually protected by the mandible above and the sternum below. Damage to the laryngotracheal skeleton occurs when either the steering wheel is forced forward and upward into the neck or when the driver's head strikes against the windshield allowing the exposed neck to collide with the steering wheel. With the head thus extended, the larynx is not only less protected, but also less mobile and therefore less likely to deflect or escape a direct blow.[7] Front-seat passengers may also sustain blunt laryngotracheal injury by falling against the dashboard. The risk of injury is greatest in motorists who are tall or have long necks. In small cars the windshield is closer to the occupant, and the risk is even greater.[8]

The laryngotracheal airway is most susceptible to injury at the three levels depicted in Figure 2. In order of decreasing frequency of injury, they are: the glottis, level of the true cords; the subglottis, below the true cords; and the upper cervical trachea, first three rings. The usual mechanism of injury is a blunt force directed anteriorly against the cartilaginous skeleton compressing it against the bodies of the cervical vertebrae.

During the physical examination, exter-

FIGURE 2. THE LARYNGOTRACHEAL AIRWAY

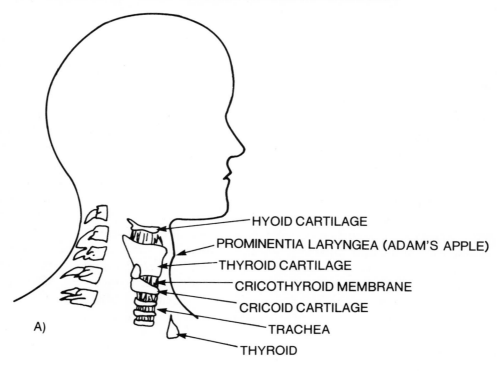

A)

HYOID CARTILAGE
PROMINENTIA LARYNGEA (ADAM'S APPLE)
THYROID CARTILAGE
CRICOTHYROID MEMBRANE
CRICOID CARTILAGE
TRACHEA
THYROID

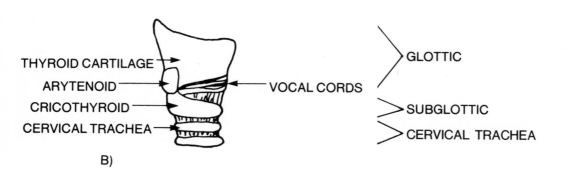

THYROID CARTILAGE
ARYTENOID
CRICOTHYROID
CERVICAL TRACHEA

VOCAL CORDS

GLOTTIC

SUBGLOTTIC
CERVICAL TRACHEA

B)

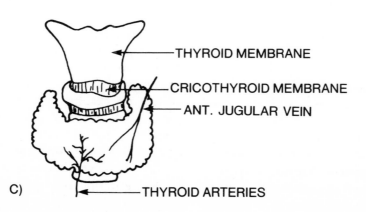

THYROID MEMBRANE
CRICOTHYROID MEMBRANE
ANT. JUGULAR VEIN

THYROID ARTERIES

C)

nal evidence of trauma and prominence of the thyroid cartilage should be noted. Palpation of the neck may disclose tenderness, loss of normal landmarks, fractures of the laryngeal cartilage or crepitance. The trauma patient with minor laryngeal injury is often hoarse without stridor and with moderate pain when swallowing or speaking. Examination of the neck may reveal either a normal laryngeal contour or perhaps a palpable fracture of the laryngeal cartilage. Signs of more significant injury include contusions or open lacerations of the neck, subcutaneous emphysema, progressive airway obstruction, loss of voice and abnormal laryngeal contour. Subcutaneous emphysema is a common finding.[9] It signifies rupture of the laryngeal or tracheal cartilage and mucosal tears allowing leakage of air. Complete laryngotracheal transsection can occur without an open wound on the neck, and sometimes in patients with minimal external evidence of trauma.

If the patient's respiratory status permits and the airway is stabilized, cervical spine films should be taken followed by AP and lateral soft tissue views of the neck and a chest x-ray. Concomitant cervical spine injury frequently occurs in patients with traumatized airways and should be ruled out before manipulation of the neck. Soft-tissue films may demonstrate fracture of the skeletal framework of the larynx, subcutaneous air, prevertebral hematoma or deformity of the air column. Chest roentgenograms evaluate possible pleural or pulmonary parenchymal damage.

Very few large series of acute trauma to the larynx and trachea have been reported and there is controversy regarding airway control using endotracheal intubation versus emergency tracheostomy or cricothyroidotomy in the management of injury.[10-13] Some physicians prefer emergency tracheostomy reporting that intubation should not be attempted because the airway is often not patent or because further trauma and distortion of the airway may ensue.[14-17] Others advocate careful endotracheal intubation whenever possible, allowing that this can frequently be accomplished without sequelae, even in patients with complete disruption of the airway.[18, 19] Indeed, recent reports have stated that after clearing the oropharynx of any debris, careful endotracheal intubation can often be accomplished without further damage to the airway. Once the endotracheal tube is in place, the surgeon has the option of repairing the trachea primarily without tracheostomy or performing tracheostomy without haste if it is necessary. When endotracheal intubation is attempted, provisions for emergency tracheostomy must be available in the event intubation efforts are not successful or precipitate airway obstruction.

In massive tracheal injuries, such as avulsion injuries extending into the thorax, endotracheal intubation or tracheostomy may not provide a satisfactory airway. As pointed out by Ecker,[20] most patients with tracheal injuries of this magnitude do not survive long enough to reach the emergency department. For those who do, cardiopulmonary bypass should be considered. It may be the only method of providing sufficient oxygenation to sustain life.[21]

CENTRAL NERVOUS SYSTEM DEPRESSION

Trauma victims may present with CNS depression secondary to cerebral injury,

16 depressant drugs, hypoxia, metabolic disturbances or shock. Even if the obtunded patient has no initial airway problems, allowing other needed resuscitative measures to be instituted, the physician must evaluate: (1) the patient's ability to maintain a patent airway over the next several hours, (2) the risk of aspiration and (3) the etiology and expected duration of CNS depression.

First rule out cervical spine injury by inspection, examination and roentgenograms. Then flex the patient's neck. If the patient resists efforts to oppose the chin to the chest or continues to move air through nose and mouth with the neck flexed, the patient's natural airway can be maintained.[22] Initially, invasion of the pharynx should be avoided. Instrumentation of the pharynx may precipitate gagging, vomiting and aspiration in the mildly depressed patient. To assess the level of consciousness, check the eyelash reflex. Gentle stroking of the eyelash will produce voluntary blinking in the lightly depressed patient. After this test, check the patient's response to verbal and painful stimuli. If the patient does not have a lash reflex, is unresponsive to verbal stimuli or responds to pain nonpurposefully, then aspiration is a danger.[23] Unless the CNS depression is quickly remedied, these patients, even without clinical airway problems, should have their airway controlled to prevent aspiration. If the duration of CNS depression is predictably short, management without endotracheal intubation may be considered because intubation itself may precipitate aspiration.

Recent articles raise serious questions with regards to the traditional therapy of aspiration of gastric contents with steroids and penicillin. These studies suggest that the administration of steroids decreases the immune response, allowing subsequent infection to occur with greater frequency, while the administration of penicillin simply selects for resistant organisms.[24, 25]

AIRWAY ADJUNCTS

Emergency medicine clinicians have numerous adjuncts in their armamentarium to maintain and protect the airway. The location of the obstruction and possible cervical, facial or laryngeal fractures should be considered in the choice of adjuncts.

Oropharyngeal Airway

The oropharyngeal airway is a semicircular apparatus, which is curved to fit over the back of the tongue and inserts into the lower pharynx. In this location, it will prevent the tongue from obstructing the airway. It should not be used in the mildly depressed patient with an intact gag reflex as it may precipitate gagging, vomiting and aspiration.

Nasopharyngeal Airway

The nasopharyngeal airway is a curved, soft rubber tube approximately six inches in length. (See Figure 3.) It should be lubricated and inserted through the nares close to the mid-line along the floor of the nose into the posterior pharynx. It functions similarly to the oropharyngeal airway. In the semi-alert patient, even with the gag reflex intact, it is better tolerated.[26]

FIGURE 3. THE NASOPHARYNGEAL AIRWAY

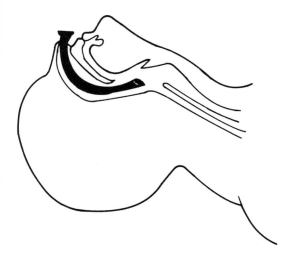

Esophageal Obturator Airway (EOA)

The esophageal obturator airway (EOA) consists of an oronasal mask with a seal, which attaches to a hollow tube with the distal end occluded. There are numerous perforations on the tube and an inflatable cuff is located just above the blind end of the tube. (See Figure 4.) The mask prevents the escape of air through the nose and mouth; the inflated cuff seals the esophagus so air cannot enter the gastrointestinal tract and gastric secretions cannot enter the airway. Oxygen is blown to the open end of the tube by a ball-valve bag mechanism, leaves the esophageal airway through the small perforations and enters the trachea, which is the only unobstructed orifice. The tube with the mask attached is passed into the esophagus blindly. Proper positioning of the tube in the esophagus is assured if adequate breath sounds are heard and the chest wall rises and falls with each breath. After checking for proper placement, the cuff should be inflated with a maximum of 35 cc of air. The EOA has been used extensively by paramedics in unconscious patients before

FIGURE 4. ESOPHAGEAL OBTURATOR AIRWAY

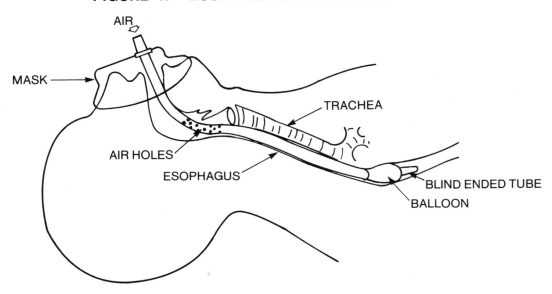

18

arriving at the hospital. Arterial blood gases (ABGs) have confirmed the efficacy of this therapeutic modality as compared to endotracheal intubation.

The advantages of the esophageal airway are that the tube can be placed quickly and "blindly" without manipulation of the cervical spine and without additional equipment, and it prevents aspiration. Potential hazards are tracheal intubation with the tube, rupture of the esophagus from excessive inflation of the tube, failure to deflate the tube before removal or retching precipitated in a semiconscious patient.[27, 28] For this reason, the tube should be used in an unconscious patient only. If a patient becomes responsive, the balloon should be deflated and the esophageal airway removed. On removal of the esophageal airway, the depressed patient may vomit. One should therefore position patients on their sides with suction readily available.

Use of the EOA is contraindicated in patients with foreign body upper airway obstruction or posterior pharyngeal bleeding. Since air is not blown directly into the lungs, the airway cannot be protected from upper airway secretions, bleeding or foreign matter. If the patient needs continued airway management in the hospital, endotracheal intubation should be performed with the EOA in place after cervical spine fractures have been ruled out. Studies have shown the EOA to be an effective way to oxygenate patients before endotracheal intubation is feasible.[29] When used appropriately, the complication rate is low.

FIGURE 5. NASOTRACHEAL INTUBATION UNDER DIRECT VISION WITH PATIENT IN "SNIFFING POSITION"

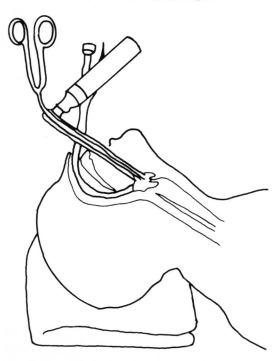

Orotracheal Intubation

Orotracheal intubation is usually the preferred means of airway control in the trauma victim, but a common pitfall is for the physician to reach immediately for the laryngoscope and endotracheal tube as a priority measure. In almost all patients after the airway has been cleansed and an airway device inserted, the use of bag and mask ventilation is the preferred therapy. This allows for the resuscitation to proceed rapidly, so that I.V. lines, physical examination, cardiopulmonary resuscitation (CPR) and cervical spine films may be accomplished while the laryngoscope and endotracheal tube are being readied.

The main advantage of endotracheal intubation is complete control of the airway. It usually protects the airway from aspiration of foreign material and allows positive pressure ventilation to be achieved with 100% oxygen. It makes the supraglottic region accessible to suctioning and eliminates the problem of gastric distension associated with mask and bag ventilation.

Prior to intubation, a patient should be hyperventilated with a mask and bag using 100% oxygen. If intubation is not accomplished within 15 to 30 seconds in an apneic patient, the patient once again should be ventilated with a mask and bag. The common errors that often make intubation more difficult are the following.[30] The first error is failure to properly position the patient. (See Figure 5.) The ideal position for intubation, with the axis of the mouth, pharynx and larynx aligned, can be achieved by extension of the head at the atlantooccipital joint while the neck is flexed at the cervical spine. Such flexions may be accomplished by elevating the patient's head with a pad. Because of the relatively large head size of infants and children, a pad is usually not required for intubation.

A second mistake is the failure to open the mouth widely making it difficult and dangerous to insert the laryngoscope blade properly. Initially, the mouth should be opened by the crossed index finger-thumb technique. If this proves difficult, the patient may be given 40 to 80 mg of succinylcholine I.V. push, to produce complete muscular paralysis within one minute, which lasts for three to five minutes. Relaxation will facilitate the intubation but during this time the patient cannot breathe or control secretions, so suction should be available. If attempts to intubate the patient fail, ventilation with a mask and bag must be continued until spontaneous respiration returns. The conscious patient must have the medication's effect explained prior to its administration to avoid a frightening experience, as the drug does not impair mentation.

The third most common mistake is improper insertion and selection of the laryngoscope blade. The laryngoscope must be held in the left hand. It is inserted from the right corner of the mouth while the tip of the blade is directed toward the mid-line. The flange of the blade prevents the tongue from obscuring the field of vision. The curved laryngoscope blade is appropriate for most adults, and is designed so that its tip should fit between the base of the tongue and the epiglottis. Because of anatomic differences, the straight blade is preferred for infants; its tip should be placed over the epiglottis.

Another frequent error is failure to expose the vocal cords properly. During attempted exposure of the larynx, the common error is to apply leverage rather than traction in the direction of the handle of the laryngoscope. The end result is inadequate exposure and broken teeth. In difficult cases, cricoid pressure by an assistant may bring the larnyx into view.

An 8 mm (i.d.) endotracheal tube is appropriate for the average size adult. For children, the proper tube is usually equal to the size of the small finger. It is important that the natural curve of the tube be preserved during intubation or it will be difficult to guide the distal end into the larynx. A malleable stylette should be used. The tube should be inserted from

20

the side or it will obstruct the line of vision. Once the tube has passed the vocal cords, the balloon should be inflated, and the lungs auscultated to insure bilaterally equal breath sounds.

The complications of endotracheal intubation include:

- Esophageal Intubation. This complication is easily detected by pulmonary auscultation immediately after tube placement.

- Intubation of the Right Mainstem Bronchus. In a recent series, this complication occurred 11% of the time and interestingly enough was often not detected by chest x-ray.[31] If the left bronchus is not totally occluded, the air that comes from the right mainstem bronchus may successfully partially ventilate the left lung. On all occasions, one should listen and make sure that both lungs are being equally ventilated and confirm the position of the tube by careful inspection of the chest x-ray.

- Trauma to the Hypopharynx or Trachea. Such a complication is usually secondary to overly aggressive intubation.

- Dislodged Tube. This complication occurs in up to 2.5 to 3.0% of the reported cases.

- Obstruction of the Tube. Thick secretions or particulate foreign matter aspirated into the lungs may obstruct the endotracheal tube. Should ventilation become ineffective, one should expect this obvious complication and either suction out or replace the tube.

- Aspiration of Stomach Content. In a recently published series, this complication occurred in 14% of tracheal intubations involving drug overdoses.[32] Thus, even with a cuffed endotracheal tube, there is significant risk of aspiration. The incidence of aspiration during endotracheal intubation is increased when the patient is hypotensive or difficult to intubate. Aspiration is associated with a definite increase in pneumonia and mortality rates.

- Pneumothorax. Pneumothorax occurs in patients with decreased pulmonary compliance who therefore require high ventilatory pressures. Frequent pulmonary auscultation and appropriate chest x-rays should alert the physician to the development of pneumothorax.

Nasotracheal Intubation

Nasotracheal intubation should be considered for the patient who is awake or who may need intubation for several days. It is also useful in the hypoxic or apneic patient with possible cervical spine injury as it avoids manipulation of the neck. The nasotracheal tube provides access to the oropharynx for suctioning and/or repair of oral injury. To accomplish "blind" nasotracheal intubation, a lubricated nasotracheal tube is passed through one nostril parallel to the hard palate. If possible, the patient should be placed in the "sniffing position." (See Figure 5.) After the tube reaches the pharynx, close the patient's other nostril and mouth so that air flow is directed through the tube only, producing an audible noise. Then guided by inspiratory air flow noise, introduce the tube further through the larynx into the trachea. If breath sounds are heard through the tube, the cuff should be inflated. If air flow stops during advancement of the tube, it has passed into the esophagus. It should be withdrawn until air flow is again audible, rotated slightly to the right or to the left and then advanced again. If the patient has a deviated septum, the tube tip will be unable to align with the epiglottis, and blind nasotracheal intubation will be unsuccessful. Nasotracheal intubation may also be accomplished under direct vision as illustrated in Figure 5. With the patient in the sniffing position, the tube is similarly passed into the pharynx. Its tip is then visualized by direct laryngoscopy and guided into the trachea using McGill forceps.

Cricothyroidotomy

Cricothyroidotomy is indicated in the depressed, apneic or severely dyspneic patient with proven or suspected cervical spine fracture, or when intubation efforts are unsuccessful. In the trauma patient, intubation may prove to be difficult with oropharyngeal bleeding which obscures the visual field, severe maxillofacial trauma or direct trauma to the larynx. If the Heimlich maneuver fails to dislodge a foreign body, cricothyroidotomy may be performed to establish a patent airway. Traditionally, the use of cricothyroidotomy has been condemned on the basis of a classic paper published in 1921, which reported increased morbidity associated with high tracheostomies.[33] However, a recent study of 655 cases of emergent and elective cricothyroidotomies puts to rest fallacies concerning this procedure.[34] Cricothyroidotomy can be used for airway control for days to weeks with an overall complication rate less than that of tracheostomies. The usual complications of tracheostomy, bleeding, disrupture of vital structures in the neck, infection, subglottal and tracheal stenosis, pneumothorax and cardiac arrest, are all less commonly seen with cricothyroidotomy.

The cricothyroid membrane is the easiest and safest site to gain airway entry in an emergency. Its location and relationship to vital structures are shown in Figure 2. A cricothyroidotomy tray should include a scalpel with a #11 blade, a trousseau dilator, a curved Mayo scissors and a standard tracheostomy tube. Although one physician can perform the operation, cricothyroidotomy is more easily carried out with an assistant. The operator steadies the thyroid cartilage between thumb and second finger of the left hand. The physician identifies the cricothyroid space with the index finger and anesthetizes the area. Then, the scalpel is inserted through this space perpendicular to the long axis of the trachea, until the trachea is entered. The assistant then inserts the trousseau dilator, following the side of the blade. The scalpel is withdrawn, and the dilator is spread. The operator uses a curved Mayo scissors to spread at right angles to the dilator. When the opening is of appropriate size, a standard tracheostomy tube is inserted. This procedure can be performed in two minutes or less.

Unlike standard tracheostomy, cricothyroidotomy is quick, can be accomplished by nonsurgeons with minimal instructions and without an operating room and has a low complication rate, which is not significantly influenced by the urgency of the procedure or the use of an operating room.[35]

22 *Percutaneous Transtracheal Ventilation (PTV)*

PTV with intermittent jets of oxygen under high pressure has been used for approximately seven years. Indications for this procedure are similar to cricothyroidotomy, i.e. for the nonbreathing patient who cannot either be quickly intubated or satisfactorily ventilated by bag, mask or mouth-to-mouth technique. A 12- or 14-gauge plastic intravenous catheter-needle assembly is inserted into the trachea through the anterior wall at some point below the larynx and above the sternal notch. Placement through the cricothyroid membrane is preferred because there are no overlying vital structures and the cricoid cartilage protects the esophagus posteriorly. To place the catheter, the cricothyroid membrane is located by palpating the transverse indentation between the thyroid and cricoid cartilages. A catheter-needle combination is attached to a syringe and directed through the midline of the cricothyroid membrane caudally at an angle of 45 degrees. During insertion, negative pressure is applied to the syringe. When air is aspirated, the needle is in the proper location. The catheter is advanced over the needle, and the needle and syringe are withdrawn. The rest of the system is then attached to the catheter.

Until recently, the catheter was connected by intravenous extension tubing to a one-way mechanical valve that attaches to a wall oxygen outlet. The intermittent jets of oxygen in the system adequately oxygenate most patients, but there is a tendency toward carbon dioxide retention

and poor alveolar washout.[36, 37] Recently, a mechanically operated device has been designed to evoke a Venturi effect causing air to be withdrawn from the trachea between the jets of oxygen.[38] The resultant active expiration phase reduces carbon dioxide build-up, and it can be constructed to mimic normal respiration. Some physicians recommend the insertion of two catheters to improve oxygenation. The complications of this procedure, which occur infrequently, include perforation of the esophagus, hemorrhage and mediastinal or more commonly subcutaneous emphysema.[39] The advantage of this technique is that ventilation can be achieved in seconds even if CPR is in progress, which may make endotracheal intubation or cricothyroidotomy more difficult. The retrograde gas flow tends to expel oropharyngeal secretions and may decrease the incidence of aspiration.[40]

OXYGENATION AND VENTILATION

If the trauma victim is apneic, cyanotic or hypoventilating in the field, the first person in attendance should perform mouth-to-mouth ventilation. This will deliver a FIO_2 of 18%, which can achieve an arterial PO_2 of 80 mm Hg. Even the alert, spontaneously breathing trauma patient should be placed on a minimum of oxygen via nasal cannula at 6 liters per minute during the initial evaluation. Although many patients ultimately do not require oxygen therapy, the respiratory and pulmonary status of the patient is often unknown, and this will provide an oxygen concentration of 25 to 40% while the patient's clinical condition is thoroughly evaluated. The use of even 100% oxygen for short periods of time will not be harmful to the patient provided the patient is under adequate observation.

In the trauma victim, oxygen exchange may become impaired very quickly. Tissue acidosis can result, and if cardiac output is decreased, tissue oxygenation may become inadequate. In cases of compromised airway, severe blood loss or shock, the patient should receive 100% oxygen during the initial resuscitation, and then on the basis of blood gases and repeat physical examinations the need for supplemental oxygen can be determined. Most initial blood gas determinations show a low PCO_2 due to the hyperventilation with a corresponding respiratory acidosis. A normal pH with a low PCO_2 is evidence of metabolic acidosis.

If the patient is conscious and breathing, 100% oxygen may be achieved through very high-flow systems that contain a reservoir bag with a nonrebreathing apparatus. The normal type of bag and mask apparatus, will not achieve a delivered oxygen concentration (FIO_2) of 100%. If the patient is not breathing, the only means of sustaining a constant percentage of oxygen flow is by use of a high-flow oxygen system, such as a Venturi mask that will deliver the same percentage of oxygen flow to the patient no matter what the respiratory rate or tidal volume. Nasal cannula, bag and mask apparatus, and nasal masks are all variable as to the percent of oxygen delivered depending upon the tidal volume, rate of respiration, the oxygen flow and the amount of room air entering the system as well as the amount of carbon dioxide the patient rebreathes. The esophagus has an opening pressure of between 18 to 30 mm Hg and any positive pressure apparatus that forces oxygen into the hypopharynx (i.e., ball valve-mask) may distend the stomach and decrease respiratory excursion.

The importance of early and frequent blood gas samples must be emphasized. It is extremely difficult to judge a patient's blood gases by observation. The patient's color is not a reliable indicator, particularly if the hemoglobin is less than 10 g%. Appreciable cyanosis requires at least 5 g% of reduced hemoglobin at the capillary level. Venous oxygen saturation seldom falls below 45%.

The trends in serial ABGs should be carefully interpreted. Under many circumstances, when respiratory failure "suddenly" appears, retrospective analysis of blood gases demonstrates that the process has been developing for some time. The fraction of oxygen in inspired gases (FIO_2) is often not adequately considered in evaluating the PaO_2. The approximate PaO_2 that might normally be expected with various levels of oxygen are listed in Table 1. Patients with chronic obstructive pulmonary disease (COPD) may be hypoxic on room air but should be near expected normal values on a high FIO_2.

If the trauma victim is hyperventilating and drops the PCO_2, remember that the PO_2 should rise by an almost equivalent amount. One method of evaluating the relationship between the PO_2 and the PCO_2 is to measure or estimate the $A-aDO_2$, which often reflects much more serious change than might be appreciated by either the PO_2 or PCO_2 alone. If the

TABLE 1

Approximate PaO_2 with Various Levels of Oxygen

FIO$_2$	Expected PaO$_2$ mm Hg*
0.21 (Room Air)	100
0.40	235
0.60	378
0.80	520
1.00	663

*Assuming A-aDO$_2$ of 10 mm Hg and PCO$_2$ = 40 mm Hg

patient is breathing room air, the A-aDO$_2$ can be rapidly estimated by adding the PO$_2$ and PCO$_2$ together and subtracting the sum from 145. For example, trauma victims may present with a PCO$_2$ of 30 mm Hg, PO$_2$ of 70 mm Hg, a pH of 7.50 and O$_2$ saturation of 93%. Most physicians would not consider these blood gases values cause for alarm. However, calculating the A-aDO$_2$ reveals an estimated value of 45 mm Hg, which is significantly above the 10 to 20 mm Hg which is considered to be normal in a young adult.[41] This may portend the development of adult respiratory distress syndrome.

Early ventilator assistance should be considered in patients with severe trauma, flail chest, shock or coma. Smoke inhalation or aspiration of gastric contents may also be indications for early ventilator assistance even if no other problems are present. Some of the laboratory indications for ventilatory assistance might include:

1. an arterial PO$_2$ of less than 60 mm Hg on room air, particularly if blood gases do not improve adequately with 40% O$_2$;

2. an arterial PCO$_2$ greater than 45 to 55 mm Hg in patients with previously normal lung functions and without metabolic alkalosis;

3. an alveolar-arterial oxygen difference (A-aDO$_2$) on room air greater than 55 mm Hg; and

4. a physiological shunt in the lungs of 40% or more.[42] Trends in the patient's ABGs and general condition are more reliable than isolated values.

Mechanical ventilators are classified as pressure cycle, volume cycle or time cycle, depending on what basis inspiration is terminated. Examples of each type are given in Table 2.[43] Pressure-cycled respirators deliver inspiration until a given pressure is reached. They fail to compensate for falling pulmonary compliance; so if the lungs become increasingly stiff, the tidal volume will decrease. The advantage of a pressure-cycled respirator is that despite a small leak, the machine will continue to cycle on until its present pressure is reached. Volume ventilators are preferred since they compensate for falling pulmonary compliance and will therefore more reliably ventilate alveoli. Intermittent mandatory ventilation (IMV) is a new technique, which allows patients to breathe independently of the respirator. With the

TABLE 2

Types of Respirators

Pressure Cycled	Volume Cycled	Time Cycled
Bird Mark 7	Bennet MA-1	IMV Hybrids
Bennet	Engstrom	Baby Bird
PR-2	Ohio 560	
Bird Mark 14	Emerson	IMV Bird

use of a one-way valve, patients breathe spontaneously when they wish. On a present time basis, a breath is delivered by the machine, and the valve closes. This allows the machine to serve as a back-up in weak patients and is also useful in weaning respirator-dependent patients.

Most patients should be ventilated with a mechanical tidal volume of 12 to 15 ml/kg body weight. This is twice the patient's normal volume, but it is necessary to avoid progressive atelectasis that occurs at lower volumes. Respiratory rates should be set relatively low, about ten to 14 breaths per minute, to avoid respiratory alkalosis. If respiratory alkalosis does develop, mechanical dead space is added to keep the PCO_2 approximately 35 mm Hg. Initially, 40% oxygen is utilized unless the patient has aspiration pneumonitis, pulmonary edema or adult respiratory distress syndrome (ARDS), in which case 100% oxygen should be utilized until blood gases are obtained. Thereafter, one should utilize the lowest FIO_2 that will generate a PO_2 greater than or equal to 70 to 80 mm Hg.

Patients with severe ventilation/perfusion derangement, as seen in ARDS, may not be adequately oxygenated even with high inspired oxygen concentrations. Patients who cannot maintain a PO_2 greater than 60 mm Hg on 60% oxygen are candidates for positive end expiratory pressure (PEEP). PEEP causes an increase in lung functional residual capacity and by so doing often improves oxygenation. Recent reports in the literature are enthusiastic regarding the utilization of PEEP for the treatment and perhaps prophylaxis of ARDS.[44-46] However, PEEP is not always beneficial, particularly if it exceeds 8 cm H_2O. In some patients, PEEP will increase pulmonary vascular resistance and decrease venous return, therefore producing a fall in cardiac output. This deleterious effect is usually seen in hypovolemic patients.[47] In patients with chronic obstructive pulmonary disease, PEEP may overexpand relatively normal alveoli instead of expanding the atelectatic alveoli. Management of these difficult patients is most easily accomplished when facilities for the measurement of functional residual capacity, cardiac output, pulmonary vascular resistance, wedge pressure and blood gases are available.

SUMMARY

Trauma is the leading cause of death in the young population, and mortality is frequently caused by respiratory failure. It is, therefore, imperative that emergency medicine clinicians anticipate and recognize respiratory problems in patients and develop an understanding of the technical aspects, indications and complications of the important airway adjuncts and respirators. The early institution of appropriate therapy could significantly increase survival rates.

REFERENCES

1. Martin A, et al: Respiratory insufficiency in combat casualties. *Ann Surg* 170:30–38, July 1969.

2. Guildner CW: Resuscitation—opening the airway. *JACEP* 5:588–590, August 1976.

26

3. Edgerton M: Maxillofacial and Neck Injuries, in Ballinger, W (ed): *The Management of Trauma.* Philadelphia, WB Saunders Co, 1973, pp 225–231.

4. Schultz RC: The management of facial fractures. *Surg Clin N Amer* 53:1 Philadelphia, WB Saunders Co, February 1973.

5. Converse J: *Surgical Treatment of Facial Injuries,* ed. 3. Baltimore, Williams and Wilkins, 1974, pp 86–131.

6. Cohn M, Larson DL: Laryngeal injury. *Arch Otolaryngol* 102:166–170, March 1976.

7. Middleton P: Traumatic laryngeal stenosis. *Ann Otol* 75:139–148, 1966.

8. Nahum AM: Immediate care of acute blunt laryngeal trauma. *J Trauma* 9:112–125, 1969.

9. Lambert GE, McMurry GT: Laryngotracheal trauma: Recognition and management. *JACEP* 5:883–887, November 1976.

10. Sheely CH II, Mattox KL, Beall AC: Management of acute cervical tracheal trauma. *Am J Surg* 128:805–808, 1974.

11. Brandenberg JH: Problem of closed laryngeal injury. *Arch Otolaryngol* 81:91–96, 1965.

12. Dowie LN: The management of open neck injuries involving the air and food passages. *St Bartholomew Hosp J* 69:186–189. 1965.

13. Munnel ER: Fracture of major airways. *Am J Surg* 105:511–513, 1963.

14. Alfonso WA, Pratt LL, Zollinger WK: Complications of laryngotracheal disruption. *Laryngoscope* 84:1276–1290, 1974.

15. Harris HH, Ainsworth JZ: Immediate management of laryngeal and tracheal injuries. *Laryngoscope* 75:1103–1115, 1965.

16. Strafe R, Boies LR: The emergency management of trauma. *Otolaryngol Clin N Amer* 9:315–329, 1976.

17. Nahum AM: *J Trauma* 9:112–125, 1969.

18. Lambert GE, et al: *JACEP* 5:883–887, November 1976.

19. Sheely C, et al: *Am J Surg* 128:805–808, 1974.

20. Ecker RR, et al: Injuries of the trachea and bronchi. *Ann Thorac Surg* 11:289–298, 1971.

21. Sheely CH, et al: *Am J Surg* 128:805–808, 1974.

22. Redding JS, Tabeling BB, Parham AM: Airway management in patients with CNS depression *JACEP* 7:401–403, November 1978.

23. Redding JS, et al: *JACEP* 7:401–403, November 1978.

24. Wolfe JE, Bone RC, Ruth EW: Effects of corticosteroids in the treatment of patients with gastric aspiration. *Am J Med* 63:719–727, November 1977.

25. Brynum LJ, Pierce AK: Pulmonary aspiration of gastric contents. *Am Rev Resp Dis* 114:1129–1137, 1976.

26. Wanner A, Zighelbom A, Sacker M: Nasopharyngeal airway: A facilitated access to the trachea. *Ann Intern Med* 75:593–595, 1971.

27. Scholl D, Hao Tsai S: Esophageal perforation following the use of the esophageal obturator airway. *Radiology* 122:315–316, February 1977.

28. Johnson KR, Genovesi MG, Lassar KH: Esophageal obturator airway: Use and complications. *JACEP* 5:36–39, January 1976.

29. Schofferman J, Oill P, Lewis J: The esophageal obturator airway. *Chest* 69:67–71, January 1976.

30. Salem MR, Mathrubhutham M, Bennett EJ: Difficult intubation. *N Engl J Med* 295:879–881, October 1976.

31. Jay S, Johansen WG, Pierce AK: Respiratory complications of the overdose with sedative drugs. *Am Rev Resp Dis* 112:591–598, 1975.

32. Jay S, et al.: *Am Rev Resp Dis* 112:591–598, 1975.

33. Jackson C, Jackson CL: Surgery of the Larynx, Trachea, and Endoscopic Surgery of the Bronchi, in *Head and Neck Surgery.* Hagerstown, Maryland, Harper and Row Publishers, 1974, chap 7.

34. Brantigan CC, Grow JB: Cricothyroidotomy: Elective use in respiratory problems requiring tracheostomy. *J Thor Cardio Surg* 71:72–81, January 1976.

35. Brantigan CC, Grow JB: *J Thor Cardio Surg* 71:72–81, January, 1976.

36. Jacobs HB: Emergency percutaneous transtracheal catheter and ventilator. *Trauma* 12:50, 1972.

37. Jacobs HB: Needle-catheter brings oxygen to the trachea. *JAMA* 222:1231, 1972.

38. Dunlap L: A modified, simple device for the emergency administration of percutaneous transtracheal ventilation. *JACEP* 7:42–46, February, 1978.

39. Smith BR, et al.: Percutaneous transtracheal ventilation. *JACEP* 5:765–770, October 1976.

40. Goldberg, A: Adjuncts for airway and breathing in *Advanced Cardiac Life Support Manual.* Dallas, American Heart Association, 1975.

41. Prys-Roberts C: Lung function in shock, in Freeman, J. (ed): *Physiological and Practical Aspects of Shock.* Boston, Little Brown and Co, 1969.

42. Pontoppidan H, Geffin B, Lowenstein E: Acute respiratory failure in the adult. *N Engl J Med* 287:743, 1972.

43. Uhl, R: Respiratory care in emergencies. *Compr Ther* 3:66–72. March 1972.

44. Kirky RR, et al: High levels of positive end expiratory pressure in acute respiratory insufficiency. *Chest* 67:1563, 1975.

45. Gallagher JT, et al: Post-traumatic pulmonary insufficiency: A treatable disease. *So Med J* 70:1308–1310, November 1977.

46. Douglas ME, Downs JB: Pulmonary function following severe acute respiratory failure and high levels of positive end expiratory pressure. *Chest* 71:18–23, January 1977.

47. Powers SR, Mannal R, Necteria M: Physiologic consequence of positive end expiratory pressure ventilation. *Ann Surg* 178:265–272, 1973.

Hemorrhagic Shock in Multiple Trauma

Robert J. Rothstein, M.D.
Assistant Professor and
Associate Director
Department of Emergency Medicine
The University of Chicago Hospitals
and Clinics
Chicago, Illinois

THE MULTIPLY TRAUMATIZED patient presents one of the most challenging problems that emergency medicine clinicians can face. To manage a common cause of mortality in multiple trauma—hemorrhagic shock—a team approach is emphasized, which includes a trauma captain, paramedics, physicians, nurses and aides. It is assumed that each emergency care team modifies the roles of the clinicians to meet its own needs; at the same time a systematic and organized effort is essential in achieving a low mortality rate.

The hemodynamic effects of an acute reduction in blood volume include tachycardia, decreased stroke volume and cardiac output, coupled with contraction of the vascular compartment to maintain perfusion of core organs. Release of catecholamines, antidiuretic hormone, aldosterone and cortical steroids results in peripheral vasoconstriction, a marked decrease in blood flow to the skin, muscles, extremities and mesenteric vascular bed, as well as

30

a decrease in urinary output, all in an effort to perfuse the heart, brain and lungs. Generalized cellular hypoxemia occurs, resulting in acidosis secondary to anaerobic metabolism. Hyperventilation and tachycardia continue, but unless the process is reversed, compensatory mechanisms will fail, leading to profound acidosis, myocardial depression and cardiac arrest.

To save the life of the patient, clinicians must intervene to reverse this process.

PATHOPHYSIOLOGY

Cellular Level

It is clear that the overt clinical signs and classical measurements of hemodynamic parameters are but crude estimates of the events occurring at the cellular level.[1] Decreased tissue perfusion as a result of early vasoconstriction or true hypotension reduces oxygen delivery to the cells. Under aerobic conditions, glucose is metabolized to pyruvate and then, further, to acetyl Co-A, which enters the Krebs cycle. Carbon dioxide is released, along with hydrogen ions, which combine with oxygen to form water. This process liberates 38 moles of adenosine triphosphate (ATP) for each original mole of glucose.

When oxygen fails to reach the cells, they are forced to undergo anaerobic glycolysis, wherein glucose is converted to pyruvate with only two moles of ATP formed per mole of glucose. Pyruvate cannot enter the Krebs cycle in the absence of oxygen and is converted to lactate instead, liberating two more moles of ATP. Anaerobic glycolysis is obviously inefficient and continued lactate forma-

tion eventually results in metabolic acidosis. Metabolic acidosis, however, is not an early sign of shock. In fact, initially, the shock state stimulates ventilation, resulting in a respiratory alkalosis. It is not until compensatory mechanisms are overcome that metabolic acidosis supervenes.

Respiration

Manifestations of ventilatory abnormalities in hemorrhagic shock include increased respiratory rate, decreased tidal volume, increased work of air exchange and increased pulmonary arteriovenous shunting.[2] Tachypnea therefore in an apparently stable patient should be considered an indication of hypovolemia unless another cause, such as chest wall injury, pulmonary contusion, pneumothorax, ruptured diaphragm or pulmonary embolus is present.

Central Nervous System

In addition to ventilatory stimulation, other central nervous system (CNS) effects are seen with hemorrhagic shock. Although coma will ultimately result from decreased cerebral perfusion, the earliest manifestation of shock may be subtle alterations in mental status ranging from confusion to uncooperativeness or even combativeness. Although hypovolemia and other metabolic derangements may alter the state of consciousness, hemorrhagic shock rarely results from head injury alone, except in the infant or in the adult with significant scalp or facial lacerations and uncontrolled bleeding. Cerebral edema as a result of hypoxemia and fluid shifts may contribute to altered mental status for prolonged periods of time.

Cardiovascular System

The cardiovascular manifestations of hemorrhagic shock are protean. The normal blood volume is approximately 70 cc/kg, and about 5 liters are in the intravascular space. Of these 5 liters, about two are in the form of red blood cell (RBC) mass, and three are in the form of plasma.[3] An acute blood loss of up to 20% of the blood volume (500 to 1000 cc) is tolerated without any significant symptoms. Tachycardia and diaphoresis may be the only obvious early signs. While perfusion pressure is maintained, cardiac output falls to about half of the normal baseline value. If blood loss continues, compensatory mechanisms begin to fail, and shock ensues.

Although an absolute blood pressure value of 80 to 90 mm Hg is accepted as one criterion for the diagnosis of shock, this is often a late sign. The blood pressure again is a crude reflection of the hemodynamics. The diastolic blood pressure reflects the amount of vasoconstriction present. Since one response to hypovolemia is catecholamine release, the diastolic blood pressure and pulse often rise in the early stages. The pulse pressure, the difference between the systolic and diastolic pressures, relates to the stroke volume and to the compliance of the major arteries, and drops early in the course. The systolic blood pressure represents a combination of the above factors. Even though stroke volume and pulse pressure may fall initially, the systolic pressure may be maintained in an effort to perfuse the heart, brain and lungs, at the expense of the skin, skeletal muscles, mesenteric vasculature and kidneys.

Although standard blood pressure measurements are crude, changes in any patient accurately reflect the cardiovascular status over a period of time. Systolic pressures obtained by Doppler, or through intra-arterial catheter, are more accurate in the face of the intense vasoconstriction that accompanies hemorrhagic shock. As hemorrhage continues beyond 20 to 25% of the blood volume, systolic pressure begins to fall. Thus systolic hypotension, in the face of suspected or obvious blood loss, is a sign of significant hemorrhage. Splanchnic vasoconstriction will result in pancreatic ischemia and the release of myocardial depressant factor,[4] a vasoactive polypeptide with a direct effect on the myocardium. This factor, along with other vasoactive substances released in the shock state, contributes to the cardiovascular collapse in late shock.

The body strives to maintain its intravascular blood volume, so that very early in the hemorrhagic process, fluid shifts begin. Although with acute blood loss, the hematocrit does not change initially, as fluid moves from the interstitial to the intravascular space and exogenous fluid is administered, the red blood cell dilution results in a falling hematocrit. The rate of extravascular fluid mobilization depends on the amount and rate of hemorrhage, and the patient's age, as well as the cardiovascular and fluid status of the patient.[5] If the hemorrhage continues, dilution of serum proteins diminishes the intravascular colloid oncotic pressure. Decreasing cardiac output produces severe tissue hypoxemia and acidosis. The resulting fall in the transmembrane potential of the cells allows intracellular leakage of sodium. Intravascular free water then passively follows the sodium and hypovo-

32

lemia is further aggravated by reversal of the fluid shifts,[6] if the shock state is not corrected.

Renal System

In acute hemorrhage, renal blood flow is decreased. The arteriolar constriction shifts blood flow to the juxtamedullary cortex from the outer cortex, thus reducing glomerular filtration.[7] This results in the release of renin, which produces vasoconstriction, and aldosterone, a potent mineralocorticoid, which enhances sodium and water reabsorption. Antidiuretic hormone is released from the pituitary in response to hypovolemia, which contributes to water reabsorption by the kidneys. Thus the initial response of the kidneys is to concentrate and decrease urine output. Well before other overt signs of shock are seen, the diminished output of urine will reflect signs of hypovolemia.

However, as hemorrhagic shock persists, renal ischemia becomes severe and renal compensation fails with resultant oliguric renal failure. Severe soft-tissue damage with hemoglobin and myoglobin release may contribute to the renal failure. Anuric renal failure, however, should be considered due to trauma or obstruction, rather than hypovolemia.

PREHOSPITAL CARE

Undoubtedly, paramedic personnel, mobile intensive care ambulances and radiotelemetry communication have had a beneficial impact on the treatment of cardiac disease. Those who are involved in the training and direction of paramedics in the field realize that prehospital care can significantly reduce morbidity and mortality from trauma as well. The old dictum of "load and go" has been propagated by those unfamiliar with the training and abilities of the talented paramedical personnel who can play a much more essential role than simply racing to the hospital.

In the field, paramedics first must direct attention to basic life support measures. Hypotension may result from hypoxemia alone, so the airway must be maintained and respiration supported with adequate oxygenation. Appropriate care must be taken if a cervical spine injury is suspected. Circulation should be maintained and pressure applied to external bleeding. Fractures must be splinted to minimize bleeding into soft tissues. A rapid assessment must be undertaken so that baseline vital signs can be obtained and an estimate of the extent of injuries made. Large-bore peripheral intravenous lines should be established and lactated Ringer's solution administered. If the peripheral veins are collapsed, time should not be wasted on multiple attempts.

Pneumatic trousers should be applied when hemorrhagic shock is diagnosed.[8] The legs should be elevated if pneumatic trousers are not available. Blood pressure below 80 mm Hg systolic is a relatively good objective indication for pneumatic trousers, although higher blood pressures accompanied by other signs and symptoms of shock (i.e., tachycardia, diaphoresis, pallor, mental status changes) also may dictate their use. The trousers can rapidly transfuse 750 to 1000 cc of blood from the lower extremities to the central circulation. In addition, they stabilize fractures and control hemorrhage of the lower extremities. Furthermore, the trousers produce distension of peripheral veins, which often makes the establishment of an intravenous line easier.

Thus stabilized, the patient should be moved expeditiously to the nearest comprehensive emergency facility for more definitive care. The balance between "stabilizing" and "wasting time" in the field is a matter of judgment that often must be left up to the physician in radio-communication with the paramedics. However, the fear that prehospital stabilization may provide a false sense of security for the hospital and emergency department personnel is an absurd argument against field stabilization.[9] If the emergency medicine clinicians work as a team, miscommunications should not occur.

EMERGENCY DEPARTMENT CARE

An efficient emergency medical services system offers a number of advantages to the receiving hospital emergency department. Radio communication with the mobile intensive care vehicle gives a warning and description of the traumatized patient. This allows the emergency department staff time to prepare consultants, ancillary support and operating room teams. In addition, initial stabilization facilitates the ensuing resuscitation.

The approach to the patient in the emergency department should be a team effort. Many departments ring a bell to alert the staff to the arrival of the traumatized patient. One person, the captain, should be in charge of assigning specific tasks. Paramedics, nurses, aides and physicians should respond to the directions of

the captain. The paramedics arriving with the patient can provide help, for example, removing clothing, applying electrocardiogram leads, as well as communicating pertinent history.

One clinician concentrates on maintaining the airway and breathing, while another focuses on the patient's circulation. One person should be responsible for taking and recording vital signs and should frequently give the captain the readings. Any external bleeding should be controlled by direct pressure, not tourniquets. Time should not be wasted suturing wounds until the patient is stabilized. In particular, blind clamping of vessels should not be permitted, as irreversible neurovascular damage may result.

There may be very few objective findings until 20 to 25% of the blood volume is lost. On the other hand, a patient who is hypotensive and hypoxemic may become combative, disoriented and uncooperative, but if physically restrained, will usually settle down as perfusion and oxygenation improve. The patient who has lost 15 to 20% of the blood volume may be stable in the supine position but have a significant ($>$10 to 20 mm Hg systolic) orthostatic drop in pressure and elevation ($>$20 beats per minute) in pulse rate when in the sitting position. The hypotensive patient should have the legs elevated or pneumatic trousers applied. Initial intravenous lines should be short, large-bore (12 to 16 gauge) peripheral lines as the rate of fluid delivery is inversely related to the length and directly related to the diameter of the catheter.

A central venous pressure (CVP) line then should be placed to monitor fluid therapy. A long line CVP may be threaded

34

via the large antecubital or femoral veins, or a shorter CVP line may be inserted via internal jugular or subclavian veins. These latter routes, as well as cutdowns on the femoral, saphenous and brachiocephalic veins, may be the only access in the severely hypovolemic patient. Care should be taken to insert all lines under aseptic conditions.

A nasogastric (NG) tube should be placed for draining gastric contents, which are examined for blood. Trauma is very likely to cause a reflex ileus, which may predispose to vomiting and ventilatory compromise, and can often be prevented with an NG tube.

A Foley catheter should be considered in most cases of trauma, but especially in hemorrhagic shock, as this is the only accurate way to monitor urinary output. It may be helpful to see if the patient can void spontaneously if there is any possibility of urethral injury. With the possibility of urethral or bladder rupture, a retrograde urethrogram should be considered before blindly passing the catheter. The initial volume in the bladder should be noted and then urinary output recorded at frequent intervals. A urinalysis should be done, looking for gross or microscopic hematuria, as well as hemoglobin and myoglobin pigments and specific gravity.

As the intravenous lines are inserted, blood should be withdrawn and sent for appropriate laboratory studies. The patient should be typed and crossmatched for a minimum of six units of whole blood and the blood bank alerted to "stay ahead" with four units on hand at all times. Complete blood count (CBC) is helpful as a baseline, but the initial hematocrit (Hct)

is the most important element of the blood count. The first Hct will not reflect the amount of blood loss initially, but is helpful in determining the extent of RBC loss as Hct values change. Serum electrolyte assay is especially important for patients on medications that might alter the electrolyte balance. Blood sugar studies are essential, and the presence of hypoglycemia should always be investigated with a one-minute reagent strip (Dextrostix®). Renal function studies (BUN and creatinine) provide more baseline information. A prothrombin and partial thromboplastin time are essential coagulation profiles, but platelet count, fibrinogen level and fibrin degradation products should be considered if consumption coagulopathy is suggested. Liver and cardiac enzyme studies also are helpful for baseline analysis. A determination of blood alcohol should be ordered when appropriate. An ECG should always be done and monitoring electrodes left in place.

Arterial blood gases (ABGs) are extremely important in assessing the pulmonary and acid base status of the patient. Blood gases should be obtained initially on room air if the patient's condition will tolerate this, but oxygen should never be withheld when necessary. In fact, high-flow oxygen by mask, nasal cannula or endotracheal tube should be given without concern for oxygen toxicity or respiratory suppression for the short period of time in the emergency department, as long as the airway can be controlled.

A concise history should be obtained from the patient when possible, and a rapid physical exam performed to assess the injury. If the patient is conscious, all procedures should be explained. Often a combative, uncooperative patient will settle down with a soothing, reassuring voice. Family members should be notified of the extent of injury and kept aware of the patient's progress.

Appropriate radiographs should be done as soon as the patient has been stabilized. A cross table lateral cervical spine film must be done prior to moving the patient's neck if cervical injury is suspected. A chest x-ray is essential after placement of central venous lines and endotracheal intubation, to rule out complications of the procedures and verify proper catheter and tube placement. X-rays may be helpful in determining the source of hemorrhage if it is not already obvious. If the abdomen is considered the source, peritoneal lavage[10] may provide the answer. Significant amounts of blood can be lost in soft tissues with long bone and pelvic fractures.

MONITORING AND THERAPY

Assessing Ventilatory Status

With the patency of the airway assured, assessment of the ventilatory status is made by questioning and reexamining the patient and by checking the ABGs. The initial response to the trauma will be a respiratory alkalosis. The PO_2 should be normal (>80 mm Hg) unless a direct pulmonary or chest wall injury has been sustained. Oxygen therapy should be adjusted to maintain a normal PO_2. If acidosis is present, significant hemorrhage

has occurred. Correction of the acidosis depends mainly upon improving cardiac output and ventilation. Bicarbonate therapy should be reserved for those in metabolic acidosis with an arterial pH below 7.20. The patient who does not hyperventilate in the face of hemorrhagic shock should be considered to have central nervous system depression, airway obstruction or damage to the chest wall or diaphragm. In the patient with chronic lung disease, CO_2 narcosis and removal of the hypoxic respiratory drive should be considered.

Endotracheal intubation and assisted ventilation should be undertaken whenever the PCO_2 begins to rise above (or even toward) normal; when the PO_2 cannot be maintained at greater than 60 mm Hg, despite oxygen therapy; when minute ventilation is less than 6 to 8 liters per minute; when tidal volume is less than 4 to 5 ml/kg; or whenever, in the judgment of the trauma captain, the effort of ventilation is too great for the patient. Naloxone (Narcan®), 0.8 mg I.V., should be given if drug-induced respiratory depression is suspected. Caution should be exercised to prevent or detect pneumothorax in patients on assisted ventilation.

Monitoring Response to Therapy

Central nervous system response to therapy should be recorded, observing parameters of mental status, pupillary response, cranial nerve function, muscle stretch reflexes, strength and sensation. It should be remembered that hypoglycemia is a possible cause of mental status alteration.

36

Monitoring the cardiovascular response is one of the most critical, and often the most difficult, of the tasks of the emergency clinician. Debate regarding choice of initial fluid therapy in hemorrhagic shock continues and cannot be resolved here. In hypovolemia secondary to hemorrhage, the blood volume must be replaced. From work by Shires[11] and Middleton,[12] we know that extracellular fluid volume loss in hemorrhagic shock is more than can be accounted for on the basis of blood loss alone. This knowledge, and other studies,[13–15] suggesting that survival is better for animals resuscitated from hemorrhagic shock with electrolytes and blood than with shed blood alone, have promoted the treatment of hemorrhagic shock with blood and either crystalloid or colloid solutions.

The argument against the use of crystalloid is that the lowering of colloid oncotic pressure leads to pulmonary edema and that colloids (e.g., albumin, Dextran) are more effective in expanding intravascular volume while maintaining the plasma oncotic pressure.[16,17] The opponents of colloid therapy feel that increased capillary permeability allows increased leakage of colloid into the pulmonary interstitium promoting further edema.[18] Low molecular weight Dextran, although effective in increasing intravascular fluid volume, has lost favor because of the risk of anaphylactic reaction, the transient increase in clotting time and the difficulty in further cross matching of blood.[19] Articles on the question of crystalloid versus colloid abound. Perhaps the most appropriate appraisal was made by Lowe et al.,[20] who found no significant differences in survival rate, incidence of pulmonary failure or postoperative pulmonary function in a randomized trial of Ringer's lactate solution alone, versus Ringer's and albumin, for the treatment of hemorrhagic shock in man. They did note that the average cost to the patient resuscitated with albumin was $540.92 compared to $4.92 for the Ringer's group.

The author's choice of fluid is Ringer's lactate for the initial resuscitation. The fear that the lactate concentration will contribute to acidosis is unfounded.[21] Fluid is administered as rapidly as necessary to maintain measured hemodynamic parameters at satisfactory levels. Obviously, this varies from situation to situation. In the patient without measurable blood pressure, but a palpable pulse, Ringer's solution should be infused as rapidly as possible in an attempt to expand the intravascular volume. Approximately twice the estimated blood loss should be replaced with Ringer's. Cardiac arrest in the volume depleted patient cannot be managed by applying external cardiac compression to an empty heart. Therefore, while lines are being established, preparation should be made for an immediate thoracotomy,[22] if the patient has suffered a cardiac arrest secondary to trauma. Hemorrhage can be controlled by isolating intrathoracic bleeding directly, or by crossclamping the aorta above the diaphragm to limit abdominal bleeding. Crossclamping the aorta commits the patient to immediate exploration in the operating room, as the abdominal organs will not tolerate this procedure for more than 20 minutes.

Pneumatic trousers can give a rapid autotransfusion of 750 to 1000 cc of blood and should always be considered in hemorrhagic shock. Remember that rapid deflation of the trousers will produce an equivalent phlebotomy, so they must be deflated slowly with adequate volume replacement. Blood should be given as soon as possible.[19,23] If the patient can be stabilized with crystalloid, it may be beneficial to wait the 45 minutes necessary to obtain typed and cross-matched whole blood. If delay cannot be permitted, type-specific, uncross-matched whole blood should be used in preference to low titer type "O" Rh negative blood. Type-specific blood should be available within ten minutes, a period during which the infusion of Ringer's lactate should suffice.

Packed RBCs offer the advantage of decreased infusion of potassium and citrate, fewer platelet aggregates and decreased risk of allergic reaction, hepatitis and other communicable diseases.[24,25] However, packed cells cannot be infused as rapidly as whole blood, and the patient may benefit from the volume and proteins in whole blood. Consideration should be given to alternating fresh with banked blood, if available, and to add one unit of fresh frozen plasma and 10 ml of 10% calcium chloride with every fourth unit of transfused blood. Fresh frozen plasma will replenish depleted coagulation factors. Although there is some question about the clinical significance of low levels of ionized calcium,[26] $CaCl_2$ is added to counteract the chelation of calcium by the anticoagulant in the banked blood. Platelet concentrates must also be considered. Repeat Hct should guide blood replacement with the goal being a stable Hct at 30 to 35%.

Autotransfusion devices should be considered standard equipment in emergency departments that deal with many trauma cases.[27] Blood lost into the intraperitoneal or intrathoracic cavities can be reclaimed, anticoagulated and filtered. The autotransfusion devices thus are capable of providing whole blood that is rapidly available and compatible with the patient's own.

Central Venous Pressure

Fluid and blood should be administered with careful monitoring.[28] Of course, the blood pressure and pulse are critical signs, but again, imprecise reflections of the underlying process. The CVP is a measurement of the filling pressure of the right heart and accurately reflects right- and leftsided cardiac volume status in the healthy heart. Therefore, in the young, traumatized victim in hemorrhagic shock, observation of the CVP along with the blood pressure, pulse, urinary output and sensorium is adequate for gauging fluid therapy. Fluid should be administered until an accurately placed, well-functioning CVP line registers pressures of 10 to 12 cm H_2O.

On the other hand, in the older patient or those with prior cardiopulmonary disease, the CVP may not adequately reflect left-heart filling and may be misleading.[29] In such cases, it is helpful to insert a unidirectional, balloon-tipped, flow-directed Swan-Ganz catheter.[30] The Swan-Ganz catheter will enable the physician with the appropriate monitoring equipment and knowledge, to make a number of helpful and often critical determinations, such as pulmonary artery and

38

pulmonary capillary wedge pressure and cardiac output.[31,32]

Patients may exhibit a high or normal CVP in the face of relative hypovolemia. In these patients, it is important to be able to monitor left-heart pressures as well, and to adminster fluid in an attempt to maintain mean pulmonary capillary wedge pressure (8 mm Hg) and mean pulmonary artery pressures (15 mm Hg) near normal.

In the absence of sophisticated equipment, the CVP alone must suffice. Fluid can be administered in the face of a high CVP (accurately positioned) if the CVP does not continue to climb, which may lead to serious fluid overload. A "reversible" fluid challenge may be given with pneumatic trousers. By partially inflating the trousers and watching the flux in CVP, one can estimate fluid status. If additional fluid lowers the CVP, indicating better filling pressure and increased cardiac output, continued fluid therapy is necessary. If the CVP rises, the fluid challenge can be reversed by deflating the trousers.

Urinary Output

Urinary output should be monitored carefully. A urine/serum osmolality ratio of greater than 1.2/1, or a urine sodium falling below 10 to 20 mEq/liter indicate diminished renal perfusion.[7] An attempt should be made to maintain urine output at 30 to 50 /cc per hour with fluid therapy. Diuretics should not be used with hypovolemia as they only aggravate the condition. If, however, low urinary output persists with adequate volume replacement, small doses (5 to 10 mg) of furosemide (Lasix®) should be administered. The dosage should be doubled if there is no response.

If a second dose still produces no urine, 12.5 to 25.0 g of mannitol may be administered while the dosage of furosemide may be doubled again (that is, quadruple the initial dose) until the patient responds or 1000 mg is reached. If still no response is seen, ethacrynic acid (Edecrin®), 100 to 200 mg may be added. Dialysis may be the only alternative if diuretics fail. Remember that acidosis may antagonize the effects of the diuretics and correction of acidosis may produce dramatic diuresis.

Vasopressors

Vasopressors should not be used in the patient who is hypovolemic. Even though the blood pressure may be artificially elevated with pressor agents, it is elevated at the expense of perfusion of vital organs. Further cellular hypoxemia and acidosis will simply compound the problem. However, if normovolemia has been established and the patient is still hypotensive, a cardiogenic contribution should be considered and rapid digitalization instituted, using half the appropriate digitalizing dose. Patients who remain hypotensive may need a pressor. The drug of choice in the normovolemic patient in shock is dopamine (Intropin®).[33] In small doses, (2 to 5 μg/kg per minute) dopamine increases renal and splanchnic blood flow without significant change in the cardiac output or blood pressure. At higher doses (5 to 15 μg/kg per minute) slight, peripheral vascular resistance develops and, with an increase in cardiac output, the blood pressure may be elevated. At high doses (30 to 50 μg/kg per minute) there is greater vasoconstriction, and cardiac output may fall. The balance is delicate.

Drugs and Medication

Epinephrine is not to be used except for treatment of dysrhythmias. Dopamine gives a more consistent inotropic response and is preferable. Isoproterenol is a potent inotropic agent, but produces peripheral vasodilatation and increases myocardial oxygen demand and may be detrimental.

Steroids continue to be controversial. Steroids will reduce total peripheral resistance and mean arterial pressure, while stabilizing lysosomal membranes and interfering with complement reaction. Although steroids may produce some beneficial effects, studies have not shown that they reduce mortality[34] with hemorrhagic shock. On the other hand, they do not seem to cause harm in the short term. If used, they should be given early and in pharmacological doses. Antibiotics should be used to treat specific infections, and tetanus prophylaxis should be administered when appropriate.[35]

If vigorous resuscitative measures have failed to produce the desired response, other correctable causes of poor cardiac output should be sought. Adequate ventilation and fluid replacement should be assured; pneumothorax should be ruled out; cardiac tamponade should be suspected as appropriate; pulmonary embolus, sepsis, adrenal insufficiency, electrolyte or acid-base abnormalities and hypothermia should be considered; finally drug interaction (e.g., reserpine or other prior antihypertensive therapy) should be investigated before a diagnosis of irreversible shock is made. Adequate resuscitation of the patient has been accomplished when the blood pressure and pulse have stabilized, acid-base status and oxygenation have normalized, sensorium is improving and other hemodynamic parameters are controlled. This does not mean, however, that the patient is "cured." Further consultation should be sought so that definitive care, when necessary, can be rendered.

SUMMARY

The approach to the patient in hemorrhagic shock should be systematic and organized in a team fashion. Immediate intervention in the form of maintenance of airway, breathing and circulation begins in the prehospital setting, but should continue throughout the resuscitation. The resuscitation should be aggressive, directed at specific causes of hemorrhage and guided by clinical and hemodynamic parameters. Fluid administered under careful monitoring is the mainstay of therapy, while inotropic agents, vasopressors and antibiotics are of secondary importance.

REFERENCES

1. Schumer W, Sperling R: Shock and its effect on the cell. *JAMA* 205:75–79, 1968.
2. Proctor HJ, Ballantine TVN, Broussard ND: An analysis of pulmonary functions following nonthoracic trauma with recommendations for therapy. *Ann Surg* 172:180–189, 1970.
3. Lucas CE: Resuscitation of the injured patient: the three phases of treatment. *Surg Clin N Amer* 57:3–15, 1977.
4. Lefer AM: Role of a myocardial depressant factor in the pathogenesis of hemorrhagic shock. *Fed Proc* 29:1836–1847, 1970.

40

5. Moore FD: The effects of hemorrhage on body composition. *N Engl J Med* 273:567–577, 1965.
6. Carrico CJ, Canizaro PC, Shires T: Fluid resuscitation following injury: rationale for the use of balanced salt solutions. *Crit Care Med* 4:46–54, 1976.
7. Hayes DF, Werner MH, Rosenberg IK, et al: Effects of traumatic hypovolemic shock on renal function. *J Surg Res* 16:490–497, 1974.
8. McSwain NE: Pneumatic trousers and the management of shock. *J Trauma* 17:719–724, 1977.
9. McManus WF, Aprahamion C, Darin JC: Prehospital advanced emergency care: A potential pitfall. *J Trauma* 18:305–307, 1978.
10. Jergens ME: Peritoneal lavage. *Am J Surg* 133:365–369, 1977.
11. Shires GT, William J, Brown F: Simultaneous measurement of plasma volume, extracellular fluid volume, and red blood cell mass in man utilizing I^{131}, $S^{35}O_4$, Cr^{51}. *J Lab Clin Med* 55:776–783, 1960.
12. Middleton ES, Mathews R, Shires GT: Radiosulphate as a measure of the extracellular fluid in acute hemorrhagic shock. *Ann Surg* 170:174–186, 1969.
13. Zollman W, Culpepper RD, Turner MD, et al: Hemorrhagic shock in dogs. *Am J Surg* 131:298–305, 1976.
14. McClelland RN, Shires GT, Baxter CR, et al: Balanced salt solution in the treatment of hemorrhagic shock. *JAMA* 199:830–834, 1976.
15. Shires GT, Coln D, Carrico J, et al: Fluid therapy in hemorrhagic shock. *Arch Surg* 88:688–693, 1964.
16. Shoemaker WC: Comparison of the relative effectiveness of whole blood transfusions and various types of fluid therapy in resuscitation *Crit Care Med* 4:71–78, 1976.
17. Skillman JJ: The role of albumin and oncotically active fluids in shock. *Crit Care Med* 4:55–61, 1976.
18. Weaver DW, Ledgerwood AM, Lucas CE, et al: Pulmonary effects of albumin resuscitation for severe hypovolemic shock. *Arch Surg* 113:387–392, 1978.
19. Buchanan EC: Blood and blood substitutes for treating hemorrhagic shock. *Am J Hosp Pharm* 34:631–636, 1977.
20. Lowe RJ, Moss GS, Jilek J, et al: Crystalloid vs colloid in the etiology of pulmonary failure after trauma: a randomized trial in man. *Surg* 81:676–683, 1977.
21. Coran AG, Ballantine TV, Horwitz OL, et al: The effects of crystalloid resuscitation in hemorrhagic shock on acid-base balance: A comparison between normal saline and Ringer's lactate solutions. *Surg* 69:874–880, 1971.
22. Mattox KL, Beall AC, Jordan GL, et al: Cardiorrhaphy in the emergency center. *J Thor Cardio Surg* 68:886–893, 1974.
23. McCurdy PR: Blood component therapy. *Postgrad Med* 62:143–147, 1977.
24. Moss GS, Saletta JD: Traumatic shock in man. *N Engl J Med* 290:724–726, 1974.
25. Johnston DA: Blood transfusion: use and abuse of blood components. *West J Med* 128:390–398, 1978.
26. Howland WS: The cardiovascular effects of low levels of ionized calcium during massive transfusion. *Surg Gyn Obstet* 145:581–586, 1977.
27. O'Riordan WD: Autotransfusion in the emergency department. *JACEP* 6:233–237, 1977.
28. Berk JL: Monitoring the patient in shock: what, when and how. *Surg Clin N Amer* 55:713–720, 1975.
29. Risk C, Rudo N, Falltrick R, et al: Comparison of right atrial and pulmonary capillary wedge pressures. *Crit Care Med* 6:172–175, 1978.
30. Swan HJC, Ganz W: Use of balloon flotation catheters in critically ill patients. *Surg Clin N Amer* 55:501–520, 1975.
31. Welsel RD, Vito L, Dennis RC, et al: Clinical application of thermodilution cardiac output determinations. *Am J Surg* 129:449–454, 1975.
32. Hartong JM, Dixon RS: Monitoring resuscitation of the injured patient. *JAMA* 237:244, 1977.
33. Goldberg LI: Dopamine—clinical uses of an endogenous catecholamine. *N Engl J Med* 291:707–710, 1974.
34. Pinilla J, Wright CJ: Steroids and severe hemorrhagic shock. *Surgery* 83:489–494, 1977.
35. Rothstein RJ, Baker FJ: Tetanus: recognition and management. *JAMA* 240:675–676, 1978.

Pathophysiology, Diagnosis and Treatment of Head Trauma

James R. Roberts, M.D.
Assistant Professor in Emergency Medicine
The Medical College of Pennsylvania
Philadelphia, Pennsylvania

IT IS IMPOSSIBLE for practicing emergency medicine clinicians to avoid confronting the problems of acute head trauma. Major brain and head injury is often feared, and shrouded in a mystique that stems from failure to comprehend basic principles of pathophysiology or failure to exercise common sense. Not all patients with head trauma require the expertise of a neurosurgeon. In fact, only 12% of patients on a neurosurgical service with head injury significant enough to produce unconsciousness require surgery.[1] All patients do, however, need careful assessment by the emergency physician, since ultimate outcome depends highly on initial observations and treatments. By the time the neurosurgeon can usually reach the hospital, the patient's clinical course has been set.

The critical tasks of delineating the extent of injury and initiating treatment fall on the emergency department clinicians. Treatment decisions must often be made without the luxury of CAT scans,

42

arteriograms or two hours of observation. It does little good to call a neurosurgeon to evaluate an unconscious trauma victim while the patient exsanguinates in the x-ray department from a ruptured spleen. Likewise, the alcoholic with a blood alcohol level of 600 mg% may die of a potentially reversible epidural hematoma while the unwary clinicians patiently wait for the patient to "sober up."

INCIDENCE OF HEAD TRAUMA

Considering the incidence of head trauma in this country, *no* emergency department can avoid treating it.[2] In 1975, ten million people, or 3.68% of the population of the United States sustained head injuries that required medical attention.[3] Almost one out of every 25 people in this country will suffer head trauma this year.

Over 50% of head injuries result from falls or direct blows.[4] Head injuries occur in 70% of automobile accidents, either as isolated injuries or as one of many injuries. Automobile accidents are the number one killers of people age 15 to 24, and two thirds of the deaths are the direct result of head trauma.[3] In 1972, 16 deaths in collegiate football were caused by acute subdural hematoma.[5] A significant percentage of the working population is disabled on any single day as a result of head injury occurring on the job.

Head injury is only one facet of multiple trauma. Serious head trauma often means serious neck trauma, since 10% of automobile accidents involve neck injuries. Over half of automobile accident victims have trauma to the lower extremities and 38% have associated chest injuries.[3] Twelve

percent of patients with head injury have been drinking prior to trauma,[1] and countless heart attacks, hypoglycemic episodes and other metabolic diseases precipitate head trauma. Such conditions may be overlooked during initial assessment unless the emergency medical clinician is alert. Because trauma may be so undifferentiated initially, unquestionably, trained clinicians should be the first to care for acute head injuries.

MECHANISM OF INJURY

Although there may be great damage to the scalp, skull and facial structures, the most critical aspect of head trauma is injury to the brain itself. The amount of energy transmitted to the brain is equal to the total force minus the energy dissipated by the disruption of the scalp and skull. Therefore a major skull injury, such as a fracture, may actually indicate less direct brain injury through energy dissipation.

Fatal brain injury frequently occurs even without the slightest evidence of skull fracture or scalp pathology. Because of the inability of the skull to expand, closed head trauma resulting in brain edema is particularly devastating. Obviously, the lack of ecchymosis, fracture or laceration in no way should deter the physician from investigating the possibility of life-threatening head trauma.

INITIAL INJURY

The extent of brain injury depends upon the type and amount of force applied to the head at the time of the impact. Direct destruction of brain substance results from a gunshot wound or other penetrating object. Alternatively, injury may result from forces transmitted to the brain in rapid acceleration and deceleration. The mechanism of injury in this case is based on inertia and momentum of the brain as it undergoes complex rotatory, deforming and compressive forces. Brain compression is extensive with deceleration, which occurs in falls or windshield injuries, although complex combinations of physical forces produce most human craniocerebral injuries.[6]

Anatomically, the upper brainstem is relatively "fixed" in the skull, and the cerebral hemispheres are likely to rotate around the brainstem during trauma, intensifying compression forces. The temporal and frontal lobes are anatomically most liable to injury, regardless of the direction of the blow, as they are flung across the relatively rough surfaces of the sphenoid ridges, free edges of the tentorium cerebelli, cribriform plate and the clinoid process at the base of the skull. Injury results from laceration, abrasion and contusion of the brain tissue, and rupture of bridging veins. By comparison, the occipital and parietal lobes are less likely to be damaged because they are surrounded by relatively smooth skull.

Injury is not limited to areas of direct trauma or to effects of skull anatomy in the contrecoup type injury, in which damage is produced at the brain-skull interface opposite the site of the application of force. Contrecoup injury may result from forcing the brain against the opposite side of the skull, but more likely, it results from a transient negative pressure produced within the brain substance at the same time a positive pressure is produced at the point of impact, causing the brain to be "pulled away" from the opposite side of the skull.

Loss of Consciousness

Consciousness has two components: (1) the content of consciousness, which is quite ambiguous and is represented by higher cerebral functions dependent on the integrity of the hemispheres, and (2) the "on-off" mechanism. Unconsciousness, or the "off" state, is due to depression of the reticular activating system of the brainstem.[7] The actual mechanism of this depression is unknown. Although no gross neuropathological changes consistently follow experimental concussion, some neuronal disruption can be seen on microscopic examination of the brainstem reticular formation.[8] Loss of consciousness bears little relationship to skull fracture and occurs most commonly in rapid acceleration-deceleration injury.

Motion of the head, especially rotation, is an important prerequisite for unconsciousness following head trauma.[9,10] If an experimental animal is struck on the head, which is held stationary by a clamp, loss of brainstem reflexes will not occur. However, if the head is freely movable, a torque effect on the upper brainstem is most easily obtainable, resulting in an almost instant neuronal dysfunction and loss of consciousness. This may explain the loss of consciousness in head trauma and how a boxer can be "knocked out" with a blow to the jaw, which produces a rotational effect. Loss of consciousness is probably not the result of a wave of high intracranial pressure or cerebral anemia.

44 The sensation of "seeing stars" following head trauma probably results from initial gross excitation of the nervous system. Loss of consciousness following head trauma should not be taken lightly, for 80% of deaths from head trauma occur in patients unconscious at the time of admission.

Concussion

Concussion is not synonymous with loss of consciousness, although most concussions involve a period of unconsciousness. Concussion is a clinical diagnosis defined as a temporary neurogenic dysfunction following head trauma from which the subject recovers in minutes to hours. Most symptoms disappear within a couple of hours, except perhaps nonspecific symptoms such as headache or dizziness which may take a few weeks to resolve. Concussion is probably related to a sudden rise in intracranial pressure although numerous etiologies have been advanced.[11] Other neurological dysfunctions resulting from concussion include drowsiness, dizziness, inability to concentrate, visual disturbances, gait abnormalities, confusion and irritability.

No gross neuropathological changes consistently result from experimental concussion, and complete recovery is the rule. Occasionally, death has occurred with no lesion found at autopsy. Amnesia for the specific event and for events preceding the trauma (retrograde amnesia) are consistently found in concussion. Although there is immediate complete paralysis of the nervous system after concussion, a normal state is regained within a few seconds to a few hours.

SECONDARY INJURY

Severe brain injury is commonly the result of secondary pathophysiological factors, including hypoxia, hypercarbia, acidosis and changes in cerebral blood flow. The final common pathway is cerebral edema and intracranial hypertension resulting in death from brain herniation.[12]

Hypoxia

Hypoxemia is present almost immediately after most craniocerebral injury. Almost 50% of patients with severe head trauma have a PaO_2 of less than 60 torr. Hypoxemia results from upper airway obstruction, CNS depression of ventilation and aspiration of secretions, blood and vomitus. It can cause profound cerebral edema, both by direct cellular response, cytotoxic edema and by vasodilatation, cerebral congestion. A minor head injury accompanied by hypoxemia can easily be converted into permanent brain damage. Therefore, all unconscious patients should be assumed to be hypoxic until an arterial blood gas (ABG) proves otherwise.

Hypercarbia

Hypercarbia is a potent cerebral vasodilator. An elevated PCO_2 increases intracranial pressure and hence, can worsen intracranial bleeding. An increase of PCO_2 to 50 mm Hg in a normal person increases cerebral blood flow by 55%.[13] Controlled hyperventilation is an important therapeutic modality in head trauma.

Acidosis

Systemic acidosis, from either inadequate ventilation or systemic hypotension, causes cerebral vasodilatation and aggravates cerebral edema. Local tissue acidosis in the brain in areas of contusion may cause local vasodilatation.[14]

Changes in Cerebral Blood Flow

The monitoring and understanding of cerebral blood flow following head trauma are probably the most significant advances in treating severe head trauma. Such monitoring is beyond the scope of the emergency department, but an understanding of the physiology is necessary for intelligent therapeutics.

An adult has an initial decrease in cerebral blood flow following trauma.[15] The degree of decrease in blood flow seems to parallel the change in mental status,[16] and a return to normal cerebral blood flow is seen in patients who recover. Patients who die exhibit a continual decrease in flow until no flow is detected. Regional flow is especially decreased in areas of hematoma or edema, suggesting a therapeutic basis for mannitol administration. Children, on the other hand, have a normal or supranormal cerebral blood flow and may be made worse by mannitol infusion. Obviously, cerebral blood flow patterns are still poorly understood.[17]

Cerebral Edema

Cerebral edema is an increase in brain volume due to high water content.[18] Mild edema produces little brain dysfunction, but severe edema is responsible for focal and generalized dysfunction as well as circulatory and respiratory failure. Simple brain engorgement, cerebral congestion, may occur with an increase in blood volume, from venous obstruction or simple vasodilatation, and is often readily reversible. Cerebral edema is aggravated by hypoxia, hypercarbia and acidosis—all of which dilate cerebral vessels and are amenable to therapy.

The most common form of cerebral edema following head trauma is vasogenic edema, characterized by increased permeability of the brain capillary endothelial cells.[19,20] Vasogenic edema follows contusion and can be massive, causing severe intracranial hypertension.

Following only a few seconds of hypoxia, all the cellular elements of the brain may undergo swelling. This type of edema is termed cytotoxic edema and is seen with cardiac arrest.

Intracranial Hypertension

Increased intracranial pressure is defined as a mean cerebrospinal fluid pressure of more than 200 mm of H_2O. It is best measured continuously in an intensive care unit and should *never* be measured in the emergency department via a lumbar puncture. Intracranial hypertension and cerebral edema commonly, but not necessarily, occur together. For example, brain edema may affect one hemisphere and cause focal neurological dysfunction despite normal intracranial pressure. Likewise, intracranial hypertension may occur with brain engorgement or intracranial hematoma without brain edema.

The treatment of increased intracranial pressure secondary to an intracranial lesion (hematoma) is usually surgical. Medical measures are needed to treat intracranial hypertension of a cerebral edema origin. It is the latter cause of increased intracranial pressure that is the greatest concern to the emergency physician.

46   *Brain Herniation*

An expanding hematoma or increasing edema would be of little significance if it developed in an arm or leg. Inside the skull, however, it generates pressure which displaces brain substances to quite specific areas. The skull is divided into three main sections. The right and left hemispheres are divided by the strong membranous falx cerebri, and the cerebellum is separated from the two cerebral hemispheres by a transverse shelf of dura mater called the tentorium cerebelli. Four types of brain herniation are regularly encountered. (See Figure 1.) First, cingulate herniation is displacement of the cerebral hemisphere and cingulate gyrus to the opposite side beneath the falx.

The second type of herniation, tentorial herniation, involves displacement of the medial portion of the temporal lobe, usually the uncus, through the tentorial incisura, resulting in predictable, progressive deterioration. With uncal herniation the third cranial nerve, which carries fibers for pupillary constriction, is compressed, resulting in dilation of the ipsilateral pupil. Also the cerebral peduncles, which carry the crossed fibers of the lateral corticospinal tract, may be compressed causing a spastic weakness of the contralateral arm and leg. If progression occurs, the uncus may push the midbrain against the opposite tentorial edge producing bilateral fixed and dilated pupils and bilateral spastic weakness, which soon gives way to flaccid paralysis. Epidural hematomas often produce the classical picture of temporal lobe herniation.

The third type of herniation involves displacement of the cerebellar tonsils through the foramen magnum, leading to compression of the cervicomedullary junction, followed by cardiovascular collapse and apnea. Lastly, brain may herniate through a skull fracture or site of craniotomy.

If a mass lesion is producing brain herniation, surgery must be expeditious. If the pathology is remedied in time, recovery is good. If generalized cerebral edema is the etiology, chances of recovery are somewhat lower. The key to proper management is recognizing the various stages of decompensation and initiating steps to minimize the effects of brain herniation.

FIGURE 1.   BRAIN HERNIATIONS

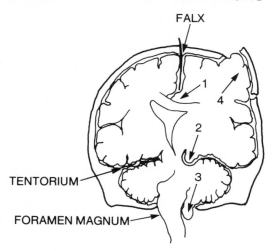

Specific sites of brain herniation: *(1) cingulate herniation beneath the falx, (2) temporal lobe (uncus) herniation through the tentorial incisura, (3) cerebellar herniation through the foramen magnum and (4) cortex herniation through area of skull fracture.*
Source: Fishman, RA: Brain Edema. *N Engl J Med* 293(14):706, 1975.

SPECIFIC INJURIES

Hemorrhage and Hematoma

Contusion and laceration are commonly seen in severe head trauma. Contusion, which implies bleeding and tissue necrosis, may or may not be associated with cerebral edema. Although contusion may be accompanied by intracranial hematoma, the injury creates a relatively fixed neurological deficit without the increasing deterioration seen with mass lesions, unless cerebral edema is severe. Generalized contusion can produce severe intracranial injury and carries a poor prognosis. The treatment of brain contusion is usually directed toward controlling subsequent increased intracranial pressure, although some surgeons advocate surgery in specific cases.

It is imperative to realize that even rapidly expanding lesions exhibit progressive neurological findings. Severely injured patients who never regain consciousness and exhibit bilateral neurological signs usually have extensive brainstem injury rather than a supratentorial blood clot, although the two entities may coexist. These patients do not deteriorate as do patients with mass lesions.

Subarachnoid Hemorrhage

Subarachnoid hemorrhage is the most common intracranial hemorrhage following head trauma. Massive subarachnoid bleeding is the most frequent finding in fatal cases, but its actual significance is unknown. In most cases, subarachnoid hemorrhage has little surgical significance because no mass effect is seen and it usually produces only a mild stiff neck or headache. Bloody spinal fluid is diagnostic. If bleeding is from a large artery death may rapidly result, and rare cases of obstructive hydrocephalus have occurred. Massive subarachnoid hemorrhage can occur without obvious contusion of the brain.

Intracranial Hematoma

Patterns of neurological dysfunction vary with the type of hematoma, but all serious lesions result in progressive loss of consciousness. Almost 50% of patients with prolonged unconsciousness have intracranial bleeding.

Intracerebral Hematoma. Solitary or multiple intracerebral hematomas may occur secondary to distortion of the brain substance. The clinical course and treatment vary with size and location. Significant hematomas may cause progressive decrease in the level of consciousness and progressive neurological deficit.

Epidural hematoma is relatively uncommon, comprising about 5% of intracranial hematomas. It is caused by venous or arterial bleeding, most commonly rupture of the middle meningeal artery or vein. Epidural hematomas are usually associated with a skull fracture and may coexist with a subdural hematoma. If the injury is of low velocity, one may obtain the classical history of a short period of unconsciousness followed by a lucid interval of a few hours; followed by rapid development of headache, vomiting and progressive deterioration, convulsions, a dilated pupil and hemiparesis, and eventual death. This particular history only occurs in about 20%

48

of patients with epidural hematomas, but the diagnosis should always be suspected when a patient suffers a fractured skull, especially if the fracture transverses a major vessel or involves the temporal bone.

The treatment is surgical removal of the clot. If surgery is performed before bilaterally dilated pupils occur, the patient has a good chance of full recovery.[21] Since this lesion may rapidly develop, causing death in hours, emergency department trephining for epidural hematoma may be justified in a patient in extremis.[22] The epidural hematoma along with the acute subdural hematoma produce a classic picture of progressive neurological dysfunction with brain herniation and death in the emergency department. Unless the physician is aware of the lesion's lethal potential, patients may be mistakenly sent home during a lucid interval or when observation has been inadequate.

Subdural hematoma is the most frequent surgically significant complication of head injury. Bleeding may be arterial or venous, and subdural hematomas are classified as acute, subacute or chronic, based on the rapidity of the development of symptoms. An acute subdural hematoma causes changes similar to an epidural bleed from which it may be clinically indistinguishable. Massive underlying brain injury is most often associated with acute subdural hematoma. Bleeding originates from cortical lacerations and tearing of bridging veins and arteries due to movement of the brain relative to its dural covering.

The chronic subdural often occurs in older patients or alcoholics. It may take six to eight weeks to become apparent and may be mistaken for other conditions, such as senility or psychosis. Most subdural hematomas are not associated with skull fractures.

Gunshot Wound of the Head

Gunshot wounds of the head merit special attention. High-velocity weapons (muzzle velocity greater than 1500 ft/sec), such as military and hunting rifles, are particularly destructive. All handguns and .22 caliber rifles are low-velocity weapons and produce somewhat less damage. Since the emergency of a missile is proportional to the square of its velocity ($E = \frac{1}{2}MV^2$), velocity is by far the most important variable. The caliber of the missile is of little consequence in low-velocity injuries. In fact, a .22 caliber handgun can create just as devastating a wound as a .45 caliber pistol, and it is difficult to correlate the size of the permanent cavity of brain destruction with caliber of the missile.[23]

Brain damage results from shock waves and from the temporary cavity which is formed by displacement of tissue from the shock waves surrounding the missile as it passes through the brain. The permanent cavity is only slightly larger than the diameter of the missile. Secondary injury results from ricochet, moving bone chips and subsequent elevated intracranial pressure, all of which occur at a greater magnitude with high-velocity weapons.[24] The path of a bullet is impossible to predict although bullets almost always completely perforate brain substance and become lodged in the skull or soft tissues of the scalp.

Although some patients may live for a short time following severe gunshot injuries to the head, only about 10% will live longer than one day.[25] An apneic gunshot victim with dilated pupils and absent brainstem reflexes should not be resuscitated unless organ transplant is considered.

Skull Fractures

A fractured skull indicates that a sizable force was delivered to the head; however, nothing can be said about the condition of the brain merely by the presence or absence of a skull fracture. As many as 30% of fatal head injuries are associated with an intact skull. Significant fractures are those that occur where underlying brain injury or hematoma formation are especially frequent, for example, the temporal bone across the middle meningeal artery or overlying the superior sagittal or occipital venous sinus. A fracture may indicate injury to the brainstem if it extends into the foramen magnum. A fracture in the sella may tear the pituitary gland resulting in diabetes insipidus, and a fracture of the sphenoid bone may lacerate the optic nerve causing blindness. Petrosal fractures can produce loss of hearing. Although a fracture may occur in any part of the skull, fractures tend to radiate to weaker parts of the skull, such as the temporal and basilar areas. It requires approximately twice as much accelerative force to fracture the skull as it does to produce a concussion.[6] The significance of a fracture is in allowing introduction of bacteria into the central nervous system (CNS) or causing cranial nerve palsies as in basilar skull injuries.

Convulsions. A fracture may be the focus for a seizure disorder if it is depressed.

Seizures commonly occur in the unconscious victim with head trauma; almost 40% of patients with a compound injury involving laceration of the brain have seizures. At the same time, seizures may occur even after relatively minor injury.

Seizures are probably the result of direct cerebral injury, such as contusion or laceration of the cortex, but intracranial hemorrhage, a depressed skull fracture, meningitis, electrolyte abnormalities, alcohol withdrawal or an underlying seizure disorder are other possible causes.

Seizures should be prevented for a variety of reasons. They not only confuse the neurological examination but they can directly harm the patient. Furthermore, post-ictal patients possess an altered state of consciousness, and postseizure paralysis can occur. Aspiration is more likely, further bleeding may be precipitated and the hypoxia of a seizure further aggravates brain damage. Unilateral pupillary dilatation following a seizure has been reported.[26] Focal seizures have been found to be accurate in lateralizing subdural hematoma and may be more reliable than eye signs.[27]

DIAGNOSIS OF HEAD TRAUMA

The emergency physician may not always be able to localize a lesion in the diagnosis of head trauma. An acute subdural hematoma may only be differentiated from an epidural hematoma by arteriogram or even craniotomy, but an expanding intracranial mass in need of prompt neurosurgical intervention must be readily appreciated.

The emergency physician must make a

50 rapid and complete evaluation of all patients with potential brain injury, not only from the neurosurgical aspect, but also from the cardiovascular, respiratory and metabolic standpoint. It is the "sorting out" of the undifferentiated patients with attention to multisystem priorities that is the art of emergency medicine.

A computer can be programed to call a neurosurgeon when an unconscious patient develops dilated pupils and a hemiparesis. The intricacies of resuscitating the critically injured patient can only be mastered by careful attention to detail and constant reevaluation, based on a thorough knowledge of the pathophysiology of all areas of medicine. Failure to look beyond the obvious precludes recognition of life-threatening conditions.

History

An unconscious patient cannot give a medical history. Since the length of unconsciousness roughly correlates with the severity of the injury and the time needed for observation, every attempt should be made to document a loss of consciousness. Many patients erroneously equate a momentary dazed condition with true unconsciousness. Eyewitnesses or paramedics should be questioned about the mental state of the patient immediately following injury. Loss of memory for events prior to the injury, retrograde amnesia, is most significant, and usually the longer the time of unconsciousness, the more marked is the retrograde amnesia.

Progression of symptoms, especially headache or confusion, is particularly important as an indicator of serious injury.

The patient who first develops symptoms three to four hours after the injury may be in serious danger. Some lesions, such as epidural hematomas, produce dramatic symptoms within a few hours. Others, such as a chronic subdural, may take weeks to become evident, often long after the initial trauma is forgotten, or minor trauma may be dismissed as unimportant by both physician and patient.

Circumstances of the injury should be sought, such as blood loss at the scene, height of a fall or condition of the wrecked automobile. If the paramedic team expresses disbelief that anyone could have survived such an accident, or that the ground was soaked with blood, the physician should be alerted to possible injury, despite a normal skull x-ray or a normal hemoglobin.

The use of medication is important to obtain. Minor head injury in an anticoagulated patient may be disastrous. In the diabetic, hypoglycemia may not only be the cause of coma but also the reason for the fall. Prior blood pressure levels will help evaluate current ones, and a drug allergy history may avert an anaphylactic reaction to antibiotics.

Alcoholism presents an especially perplexing situation. Not only is a drunk patient difficult to evaluate, but alcoholics frequently fall, may have impaired blood clotting ability, suffer from alcoholic hypoglycemia and are always in a hurry to leave the emergency department. Cerebral atrophy may produce a partially suspended brain making bridging cortical veins more vulnerable to injury. The drunk patient with head trauma deserves a second look.

Laboratory Findings

All metabolic causes of coma should be considered in patients unconscious with head trauma: drugs, hypoglycemia and alcohol intoxication as well as rarer entities such as hypercalcemia or carbon monoxide poisoning.

Routine laboratory studies include a complete blood count (CBC), electrolytes, BUN, glucose and a drug screen. Serum osmolality should be ordered if mannitol is to be given. If blood alcohol levels are not available, osmolality should be checked; if the measured osmolality is 15 milliosmoles greater than the calculated osmolality, the difference may be due to alcoholism. The single most important laboratory test that should be done on *all* serious head trauma patients is ABG analysis. All patients should be considered to be hypoxic and hypercarbic until the laboratory proves otherwise.

Physical Examination

The sine qua non of head injury management is careful and repeat physical examination, looking for subtle changes in vital signs and neurological function. All patients should have initial vital signs recorded, including temperature, with repeat measurements prior to discharge. Blood pressure should be noted in both the supine and erect position, if possible. A drop in blood pressure of 20 mm Hg or a rise in pulse rate of 20 beats per minute upon standing represents a positive tilt test and suggests hypovolemia. Shock should initially *never* be considered the result of head injury alone except in an infant whose significant blood loss may be

sequestered in a subdural hematoma. Shock can be seen if there is massive blood loss from a scalp laceration or immediately prior to death from brain herniation in either an infant or an adult.[28] Shock with head trauma should always alert the physician to a possible spinal cord injury producing spinal shock. A rapid rise in blood pressure associated with a bradycardia following head trauma (the classical Cushing reflex) signals intracranial hypertension. However, this combination is usually absent in supratentorial mass lesions unless bleeding is massive and sudden. When present, hypertension with bradycardia is an ominous sign.

Respiration is sensitive to changes in intracranial pressure, and an understanding of changes in respiratory patterns is essential to accurate assessment of a deteriorating patient.[8] Respiration is usually depressed as intracranial pressure rises. An increased respiratory rate should prompt one to look for hypoxia, hypercarbia, shock or aspiration. Irregular respirations of the Cheyne-Stokes variety signify diffuse intracranial hypertension or a metabolic disease as opposed to an isolated mass lesion. Cheyne-Stokes breathing is often a sign of impending transtentorial herniation. With brain compression secondary to herniation, the sustained, regular, rapid breathing of central neurogenic hyperventilation is seen. Completely irregular ataxic breathing is noted in the preterminal state. Complete respiratory arrest may be seen as a primary entity in some form of severe head trauma. The above pattern of respiratory changes signifies progressive deterioration.

Hyperthermia is an unfavorable prog-

52

nostic sign in head trauma, which is associated with deterioration and a rise in intracranial pressure. Hyperthermia should be controlled vigorously since it produces increased metabolic demands on the brain and can worsen cerebral edema.[29]

Neurological Examination

A normal neurological examination is a reliable factor in predicting a favorable outcome in head trauma.[30]

LEVEL OF CONSCIOUSNESS

The single most important indication of the severity of head trauma is the level of consciousness. Progressive deterioration of consciousness is the hallmark of increasing intracranial pressure. Obviously, trends in the level of consciousness must be evaluated on repeated observations; if the same observer cannot do this, either due to a change of shift or transfer to the floor, precise descriptions must be recorded.

The words stuporous, comatose or obtunded are useless since they convey only abstract ideas. A specific description of the patient's thought processes is needed, such as "patient felt it was 1945" or "the president is Richard Nixon." Alertness may be evaluated by giving the patient an instruction to "touch the right ear with the left hand, close the left eye and stick out the tongue." Such directions are preferable to tests which measure intellectual function, such as serial seven subtraction, which even physicians find difficult. Correct performance of such complex instructions, which may be repeated once, is a concrete sign of alertness. Likewise, motor and sensory func-

tion can be tested by having patients hold out their hand and close their eyes, while checking for drift. Proper performance of this test requires understanding of directions, proprioception and motor strength; subtle abnormalities can be appreciated more easily than by testing the strength of a handgrip. An awake patient should also be tested for response to pinprick and ability to coordinate extremities, with such tests as finger-nose-finger following, ability to walk a straight line and running the heel down the opposite shin.

Consciousness cannot be tested in an unconscious patient, but certain guidelines are helpful. Restlessness, agitation and combativeness are common symptoms of brain injury but may also be due to hypoxia, a distended urinary bladder, shock, pericardial tamponade or associated long-bone or rib fracture. Most importantly, they may signify an expanding intracranial mass. Agitation in a previously quiet patient needs immediate evaluation, *not* sedation.

Testing the response to painful stimuli is the most important part of the examination of an unconscious patient. Responses should be recorded in detail. "Responds to pain" tells nothing, but "withdraws right leg on pinching the right toe" is quite descriptive and reproducible by subsequent examiners. Purposeful movements, such as withdrawal from pain or pushing a pain-producing hand away indicate less CNS depression than nonpurposeful motion, such as decerebration. Decerebration, which is opisthotonos with the extension of all extremities and internal rotation of the arms and legs following noxious stimulus, signifies extensive brainstem damage that is usually irreversible.[8]

CRANIAL NERVES

Cranial nerve examination should be done in all patients with head injuries. Fractures at the base of the skull may result in cranial nerve dysfunction. Specifically loss of smell (anosmia), all degrees of blindness, facial paralysis and hearing deficits may occur depending on the site of fracture and nerve injury. Although anosmia may be permanent, temporary loss of smell is not uncommon following minor head injuries.

EYE SIGNS

A dilated pupil following head trauma is significant. If a patient is awake and alert following trauma, a dilated pupil is *not* due to increased intracranial pressure and may signal a glass eye, the use of eye drops or local eye trauma. Nonspecific trauma to the third cranial nerve may produce a dilated pupil in an awake patient, or a unilateral, dilated pupil may result from a seizure.

A dilated pupil secondary to intracranial hypertension is produced by the temporal lobe herniating through the tentorium, compressing the ipsilateral oculomotor nerve. This mechanism is always associated with a decreased level of consciousness, almost always unconsciousness. Dilation occurs first, followed by the more significant lack of response to light. Pupil dilation occurs on the same side as the subdural hematoma in 80% of cases;[27] however, this is not always the case. If both pupils become fixed and dilated, mortality rates are around 85%. If decerebral rigidity is also present, mortality rates are near 95%. If pupils are fixed and dilated for longer than 30 minutes, survival is extremely rare. Of course, dilated fixed pupils are also seen with anoxia, such as cardiac arrest, and are not always related to brain herniation. Drugs used in resuscitation, such as epinephrine, atropine and dopamine, may produce bilateral dilated pupils. Papilledema rarely develops in the emergency department, and although funduscopic examination should be done, pupils should *not* be dilated to obtain a better view.

In unresponsive patients, integrity of the brainstem may be tested by the oculocephalic reflex (Doll's eye) and oculovestibular reflex (cold caloric); their absence indicates severe injury.[8] To elicit the Doll's eye reflex, first be certain that no cervical spine injury exists. With the patient's eyes held open, rapidly turn the head from side to side. A normal reflex is for both eyes to move in a direction opposite to the movement of the head. This test is of no value in the awake patient, who, of course, has an intact brainstem, because the reflex disappears if the eyes are voluntarily fixed.

The cold caloric test is done with the head elevated 30° to the horizontal. Twenty milliliters of ice water are instilled into the ear by a catheter *gently* placed near the eardrum. With an intact reflex, the eyes move toward the side of instillation. Only in the awake patient is this deviation followed by nystagmus toward the midline. The presence of nystagmus may be used to detect malingering.

LEAKAGE OF CEREBRAL SPINAL FLUID
AND BLOOD

Blood or fluid coming from the ear, the nose or behind the tympanic membrane should alert the physician to a probable skull fracture. Such fractures may involve

54 the base of the skull and are often not demonstrated by routine x-ray.

Fractures of the temporal bone usually involve the middle ear or the posterior-superior portion of the external canal. If the tympanic membrane is intact, blood or cerebrospinal fluid (CSF) may remain behind the drum. If it is torn, blood will flow into the canal. These fractures may also involve the facial nerve or affect hearing. Ear canals should not be irrigated or blocked with cotton. Wax may be differentiated from dried blood by dipstick testing of a sample obtained with a curette. Bedside tests to identify CSF that is mixed with blood are misleading. A finding of concentric rings of blood and CSF when the mixture is placed on filter paper is *unreliable* and should not be used. Contrary to some texts, clear fluid from the nose that is positive for glucose on a dipstick is *not* diagnostic of CSF since nasal secretions are often high in glucose.[31]

Most cerebrospinal fluid leaks close spontaneously within two weeks. Surgery is rarely required unless there is displacement of bone or the leakage persists.

Ecchymosis over the mastoid area in the absence of direct trauma to the ear is diagnostic of a fracture of the temporal bone (Battle's sign), and may take a few hours to develop. Bilateral medial orbital ecchymosis (raccoon eyes), in the absence of a broken nose, is good evidence for an anterior basal skull fracture.

X-Rays

The most important x-ray in major head injury is the lateral cervical spine film. However, it is absurd to think that all skull fractures can be diagnosed by physical examination so x-rays of the skull should be taken if any reasonable chance of fracture or major intracranial injury exists. Certainly almost half of all skull x-rays currently performed can safely be eliminated. To reduce x-ray exposure[32] and to contain rising medical costs, the necessity of skull x-rays has been extensively reviewed.[33-36]

Radiographical examination of the skull following trauma is indicated by certain aspects of both the history and the physical examination.[34] Indications in the history include: (1) unconsciousness; (2) gunshot wound or other penetrating injury; (3) previous craniotomy with a shunting tube in place; and (4) injury necessitating admission or observation for over four hours. Physical examination criteria include: (1) palpable skull defect or visual conformation through a laceration; (2) CSF or bleeding (without signs of direct trauma) from the nose or ear; (3) Battle's sign or raccoon eyes; (4) unconsciousness; and (5) focal neurological signs, including seizures, hemiparesis or pupillary abnormalities.

The abuse of skull films is widespread, and the films often take the place of a careful history and physical examination. Death from head injury is common without x-ray evidence of skull fracture. Skull fractures were reported in less than 2% of patients x-rayed in one outpatient series.[35] The British literature reports never finding a case in which failure to request a skull x-ray was found to be negligent.[36] Certainly, a skull x-ray is not warranted with minor trauma, such as banging the head on a table or a child with a scalp hematoma, when the physical examination is negative and the patient is asymptomatic. An x-ray should *never* be used to determine whether or not a patient should be discharged.

A special warning is added about penetrating trauma. Pencil points, which are visible on x-rays, can cause abscess, and lawnmowers are notorious for propelling objects at high speed. Rakes, screwdrivers and children's toys also are potentially dangerous. An x-ray should be obtained to determine depth of penetration before removing an impacted object.

Depressed fractures produce a white line on the film, and this radiodensity may elude the physician unless tangential views to the area in question are obtained. The presence or absence of a skull fracture rarely influences the initial treatment, and x-rays may be deferred until a patient is cooperative enough to obtain useful films. Valuable time is often wasted in the x-ray department, attempting to obtain perfect skull films.

Fractures of the base of the skull frequently cannot be identified on routine views and the diagnosis must be inferred by physical exam. Some subtle radiographical findings diagnostic of a basilar skull fracture are: (1) an opaque mastoid sinus, (2) opacity or air fluid level in the sphenoid sinus or (3) pneumocephalus.

Many patients do not possess a calcified pineal gland, but if it is present it may be helpful in diagnosing midline shift from an expanding hematoma.

Ancillary Diagnostic Tests

Computerized axial tomography and cerebral arteriography provide the most accurate diagnosis of traumatic neurosurgical lesions, but they require trained personnel, time to perform and a cooperative or anesthetized patient. The echoencephalogram is a safe, noninvasive test which identifies a midline shift. False positives and negatives are seen, and bilateral lesions or generalized cerebral edema may not produce a midline shift. The electroencephalogram and brain scan are of no real value in acute diagnosis, but the EEG can be used to evaluate brain death in organ transplant cases. Lumbar puncture is contraindicated in the presence of obvious head trauma because of the danger of iatrogenic herniation.

TREATMENT

The treatment of head trauma begins at the accident when proper attention is paid to hypoxia, bleeding, associated trauma and cervical spine injury. All patients should arrive in the emergency department receiving supplemental oxygen and immobilization of the cervical spine. Once the patient arrives at the emergency department, rapid neurological, cardiovascular, respiratory, and metabolic assessment is mandatory. Prompt neurosurgical evaluation of critical patients is of prime importance and certainly the neurosurgeon should be consulted long before the skull films are developed. It has been shown that, in approximately half of patients dying from head trauma, avoidable complications contributed to the fatal outcome.[37] The main avoidable factor was delay in treating intracranial hematomas, caused by delay in neurosurgical consultation.

56   *Treatment of the Unconscious Patient*

Positioning. An unconscious patient, lying on the back, should initially be considered to have an obstructed upper airway, not only from the tongue but also from secretions, blood and vomitus. Unless the patient is intubated or has an unstabilized cervical spine injury, the proper position is lying on the stomach or side, with the face dependent.[38] All moving should consist of rolling the patient like a log with slight cervical traction and the head in neutral position.

Airway and Breathing. All unconscious patients should be considered to have inadequate respiratory exchange until proven otherwise. With proper care given to cervical spine injuries, *all* unconscious patients should have the trachea intubated, preferably by the blind nasal route, or over the fiberoptic bronchoscope, and a cuff inflated. The esophageal obturator airway is an alternative, especially in the field or in the emergency department, if neck injury makes tracheal intubation impossible.

The patient should be hyperventilated to a rate of 20 to 25 per minute and given 100% oxygen until blood gas determination is possible. Hyperventilation may be instituted in the field. Arterial blood gas analysis is the first laboratory test that should be considered.

Shock should be treated vigorously, as if head trauma did not exist. Bleeding should be stopped by direct compression; fractures should be splinted. All patients should have an I.V. started, but fluid replacement should *never* be 5% dextrose in water. Blood loss is treated with blood replacement.

In a normotensive patient, meticulous care should be taken to avoid overhydration, and no more than 500 cc of fluid should be given in the emergency department. Overhydration intensifies cerebral edema. The ideal isotonic solution that has the least effect on intracranial pressure is 2.5% glucose in 0.45 normal saline. Vital signs should be taken, an accurate neurologic check-off sheet should be kept and a coma score sheet may be started. Failure to use predesigned check sheets leads to short cuts and omissions in observation techniques. If the patient is deteriorating, the head should be shaved in preparation for surgery, and the operating room should be alerted.

Convulsion. All unconscious traumatized patients, especially those with compound injuries, should receive seizure prophylaxis. Sodium diphenylhydantoin (Dilantin®), by the intravenous route, is the drug of choice.[38] An adult should receive 1000 mg, 250 mg every 30 minutes, given at a rate of 50 mg per minute. Children require 10 mg/kg as a loading dose. Occasional hypotension or supraventricular arrhythmias may develop, but Dilantin® is a relatively safe drug and is preferred because it does not significantly depress consciousness or respiration.

Breakthrough seizures should be treated with diazepam (Valium®) 5 mg per minute as needed. Sodium amobarbital (Amytal®) at a dose of 100 mg per minute up to 500 mg is also a good choice.

Antibiotic Therapy. Basilar skull fractures, penetrating injuries and open fractures require antibiotic therapy that penetrates the blood-brain barrier. High-dose penicillin and ampicillin are reasonable choices. In a patient with a possible allergy, chloramphenicol is an excellent choice.

Treatment of the Conscious Patient

Vital signs should be taken immediately and a neurological check-off list ("neurowatch") should be completed. All vital signs should be repeated before the patient is discharged.

Scalp wounds are commonly encountered in the emergency department. Anatomically, the scalp can be divided into three distinct layers. (See Figure 2.) The skin, superficial fascia and galea can be considered as one layer since they tightly adhere to each other. Scalp wounds will not gape open unless all three layers have been transversed. Tough, fibrous subcutaneous fascia limits the spread of infection but aiso hinders the retraction of the numerous anastomosing blood vessels, allowing for profuse hemorrhage in simple scalp laceration.

The galea is the aponeurosis of the frontalis and occipitalis muscles, and beneath the galea is an area of loose areolar tissue, which is a potential space for blood clots to develop. This area contains emissary veins which empty into the venous sinuses and is an area for potentially dangerous infections to develop and spread into the brain. The third layer is the thin periosteum which can easily be stripped from the skull, and is often mistaken for the galea by the inexperienced.

Since most of the vessels transverse the outer scalp layer, bleeding can be controlled by either direct pressure or by a hemostat which grasps the galea and is reflected over the skin. It is folly to attempt to tie off bleeding vessels in scalp lacerations, which only leads to more hemorrhage.

All scalp wounds should be explored with a gloved finger looking for a fracture or foreign body. A common error of

FIGURE 2.   LAYERS OF THE SCALP

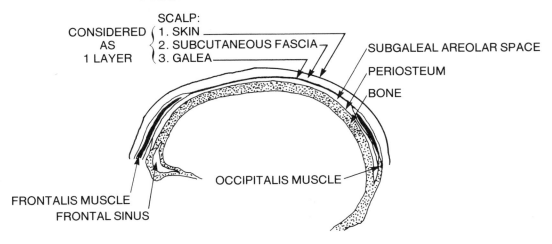

SCALP:
CONSIDERED { 1. SKIN
AS { 2. SUBCUTANEOUS FASCIA
1 LAYER { 3. GALEA

SUBGALEAL AREOLAR SPACE
PERIOSTEUM
BONE

OCCIPITALIS MUSCLE

FRONTALIS MUSCLE
FRONTAL SINUS

58 palpation is to mistake a rent in the soft tissue of the scalp for a fracture so suspected fractures must be visualized. It is reasonable to extend a laceration if the diagnosis of skull fracture is questionable. Direct visualization and palpation of the skull will demonstrate small fractures not visible on x-ray. The liberal use of lidocaine with epinephrine will facilitate examination of lacerations.

After hemostasis is obtained, the area around the laceration should be widely shaved and the wound copiously irrigated. Surrounding hair can be kept out of the way by tape or vaseline. All debris should be removed, a frequent omission. Bone chips should never be removed; they signal a need for repair in the operating room.

Severely contused tissue should be removed by sharp debridement. Often a messy stellate contusion-laceration can be converted to a clean elliptical wound. If the galea can easily be closed separately, it should be sutured with interrupted nonabsorbable sutures. The outer three layers, including the galea, can be closed with full-thickness, through and through 3–0 silk sutures tied tightly for hemostasis. Bandages are not used, and the patient can gently wash the hair 12 hours later. Scalp wounds rarely become infected.

A special caution should be made about subgaleal hematoma and abscess. Blood clots in the subgaleal area should be removed *before* the scalp is sutured, but they tend to recur if hemostasis is inadequate and may become infected. Secondary subgaleal hematomas are often large and take weeks to resolve. Without infection, they are best left alone. Puncture wounds and direct inoculation of bacteria may result in a rapidly spreading infection of the subgaleal space,[39] a serious complication that should be aggressively treated in the hospital.

Observation. The wise physician will be very liberal with the observation ward when dealing with head trauma. Some hospitals have a policy that any patient who has lost consciousness is admitted for 24-hour observation. If a patient exhibits *any* sign of a depressed consciousness, a minimum four- to six-hour observation period is needed. This can be done in the emergency department if facilities exist for true observation. A check-list should be accurately kept and reviewed at least every hour. If any sign of deterioration occurs, action is needed. Particularly negligent times for observation are at change of shift.

During the observation period, sedatives or narcotics are not given. Patients are *not* discharged with severe headache, vomiting, unstable gait, drowsiness or if they are drunk. *All* patients who have been observed and sent home should be reevaluated in 24 hours. It is wiser to keep patients in the emergency department overnight rather than send them home alone. Head trauma instruction sheets are a good idea but cannot be read by unconscious patients.

It is common for the effects of concussion to persist for a few days to a few weeks. Effects include nonspecific dizziness, balance or visual disturbances, lack of concentration, irritability and especially dull headaches. Treatment is difficult and usually consists of analgesics and possibly mild sedation. Anecdotally, short-term low-dose steroid treatment may also be beneficial.

The Medical Management of Intracranial Hypertension

It is obvious from recent work[15,16] that cerebral blood flow, intracranial hypertension and brain metabolism following head trauma are extremely complex and incompletely understood. Efforts to treat acutely ill patients on any extended basis will probably ultimately depend on continuous monitoring of regional cerebral blood flow and intracranial pressure.[40-42] There are, however, certain guidelines which the emergency physician can follow. It is best to correlate emergency department treatment with the views of the neurosurgical department in individual institutions, since the optimal therapy is controversial.

In the event of a deteriorating patient and no available neurosurgeon, the following points may be helpful.

Hyperventilation. Respiratory alkalosis reduces cerebral circulation, and there is little doubt that hyperventilation will decrease intracranial pressure for short periods of time. The beneficial effects of long-term hyperventilation are less clear. Reducing cerebral blood flow theoretically can be dangerous if patients have marginal flow to begin with, such as the elderly. Hyperventilation can begin in the field with an esophageal airway. The PCO_2 should be kept between 25 to 30 torr.[43]

Corticosteroids. The role of steroids in the treatment of traumatic injuries is unclear. Dexamethasone is the steroid that is presently most popular because of lower sodium retaining properties. High-dose dexamethasone does reduce vasogenic cerebral edema in brain tumors, but there is not always a sustained effect. Early work[44,45] demonstrated no statistically significant difference in outcome in patients treated with steroids. Recently a reduction in mortality rate from 57% in nonsteroid treated patients to 30% in patients treated with low-dose steroids and 18% in patients treated with high-dose steroids has been reported.[46,47] These figures are impressive and encouraging. Low dose therapy consists of a 10 mg bolus of dexamethasone followed by 4 mg every six hours. High dose therapy is a 100 mg bolus repeated in six hours, followed by 4 mg every six hours.

The disadvantage of steroid treatment is that fluid and electrolyte balance is much more difficult, and careful fluid management in patients is essential. Other side effects of steroids are well known. At the present time, high-dose dexamethasone therapy in severe cerebral edema secondary to head trauma seems warranted and should be started early in the course of emergency department therapy.

Osmolar Agents and Diuretics. Initially, mannitol creates an osmotic gradient between the brain and the blood. This results in a shift of water which produces a decrease in brain volume and intracranial pressure. The effect is short lived, however, since the solute reaches an equilibrium in brain tissue. Since there is a focal vasogenic edema in areas of trauma, the solute is not excluded from this edematous tissue, and in fact, probably concentrates in this area. The final result, which

60 occurs in three to four hours, is a "rebound effect" and worsening of cerebral edema unless increasing concentrations of mannitol are given. One now has to deal with the dangers of the hyperosmolar state.[48] One can document an increase in cerebral blood flow of nearly 50% shortly after mannitol infusion[49] with a subsequent increase in bleeding being noted during craniotomy.

If a patient is rapidly deteriorating, mannitol is justified to "buy time" until neurosurgery can be done, and its further use can best be determined by intracranial pressure monitoring. Mannitol can be given as a bolus of 0.25 to 1.0 g/kg or as an infusion of a 20% solution to run 500 cc over 20 minutes.[50] Furosemide and ethacrynic acid have also been used to dehydrate the brain.[51]

Barbiturates. Encouraging work has been done to evaluate the role of barbiturate therapy in reducing intracranial pressure.[52] Not only may barbiturates "protect" the brain by lowering metabolism, they have been used successfully to reduce intracranial pressure when other therapy has failed. They hold promise for the future.

HEAD TRAUMA IN CHILDREN

Children tolerate brain injury much better than adults. It is well known that head trauma is associated with a much better outcome in children who have injuries similar to adults.[53] For example, the mortality rate in adults with decerebrate posturing is about 70% but only 17% in children.[45] Bilateral unreactive pupils correlate with a 91% mortality rate in adults and 20% in children.

Children are much more likely to vomit and become drowsy following even minor head trauma, but complete recovery is rapid. Recovery is sometimes rapid enough to be embarrassing to the physician who made arrangements for hospital admission of a child who is now running around the emergency department. For this reason, resuscitation of seemingly hopeless cases in children should be pursued.

SUMMARY

A reasonable understanding of the vagaries of acute head trauma is required of all emergency medicine clinicians. The devastating potential of head injury allows one to merely start an I.V., get skull x-rays and wait for the neurosurgeon to arrive. Successful outcome requires a high index of suspicion of associated pathophysiology, a careful and continual physical examination, and early and aggressive treatment of reversible conditions. The initial evaluation and treatment of acute head injuries is clearly in the curriculum of emergency medicine, and although the problems are often complex they are not inscrutable.

REFERENCES

1. Walt AJ, Wilson RF: Some considerations in the initial management of injuries to the head and spine, in Thomas LM, Gurdjian ES (eds.) *Management of Trauma: Pitfalls and Practice*, Philadelphia, Lea and Febiger, 1975, chap 14.
2. National Safety Council: Accident Facts, 1968–1977.

Chicago 1977.

3. Jennett B, Teasdale G, Galbraith S, et al: Severe head injuries in three countries. *J Neurol Neurosurg Psychol* 40:291, 1977.

4. Schneider RC: *Head and Neck Injuries in Football,* Baltimore, Williams and Wilkins, 1973, p 279.

5. Gurdjian ES, Hodgson VR, Thomas LM, et al: Impact head injury—mechanism and prevention. *Gen Pract* 37:78, 1968.

6. Gurdjian ES, Gurdjian ES: Acute head injuries. *Surg Gynecol Obstet* 146:805–820, May 1978.

7. Foltz EL, Schmidt RP: The role of the reticular formation in the coma of head injury. *J Neurosurg* 13:144–154, 1956.

8. Plum F, Posner JB: *Diagnosis of Stupor and Coma* ed 2. Philadelphia. FA Davis Co, 1972.

9. Schwartz SF (ed): *Principles of Surgery.* New York, McGraw-Hill, 1969, p 1493.

10. Thorn GW, et al (eds): *Harrison's Principles of Internal Medicine,* ed 8. New York, McGraw-Hill, 1977, chap 335.

11. Gurdjian ES, et al: Studies on experimental concussion. *Neurol* 4:674–681, 1954.

12. Miller JD, Becker DP, Ward JD, et al: Significance of intracranial hypertension severe head injury. *J Neurosurg* 47:503, 1977.

13. Shenkin HA, Novack P: Clinical implications of recent studies on cerebral circulation in man. *Arch Neurol Psychiat* 71:148–159, 1954.

14. Gotah F, Tazaki Y, Myers JS: Transport of gases through brain and their extravascular vasomotor action. *Exp Neurol* 4:484–458, 1961.

15. Bruce DA, Langfitt TW, Miller JD, et al: Regional cerebral blood flow, intracranial pressure, and brain metabolism in comatose patients. *J Neurosurg* 38:131, 1973.

16. Langfitt TW, Obrist WD, Gennarelli TA, et al: Correlation of cerebral blood flow with outcome in head injured patients. *Ann Surg* 186:411, 1977.

17. Maurice-Williams RS: Temporal lobe swelling: A common treatable complication of head injury. *Brit J Surg* 63:160–172, March 1976.

18. Fishman RA: Brain edema. *N Engl J Med* 293:706–711, 1975.

19. Klatzo I, Seitelberger F: *Brain Edema.* New York, Springer-Verlag, 1967.

20. Manz AJ: The pathology of cerebral edema. *Hum Pathol* 5:291–313, 1974.

21. Hooper R: Observation on extradural hemorrhage. *Brit J Surg* 47:71, 1959.

22. Committee on Trauma of the American College of Surgeons: Head Trauma, in *Early Care of the Injured Patient* ed 2. Philadelphia, WB Saunders Co., 1976,

chap 8.

23. Kirkpatrick JB, DiMaio V: Civilian gunshot wounds of the brain. *J Neurosurg* 49:185–198, 1978.

24. Adeloge A: Mortality in missile wounds of the head. *Brit J Surg* 59:201–205, 1972.

25. Freytag E: Autopsy findings in head injuries from firearms. *Arch Pathol* 75:215, 1963.

26. Pant SS, Benton JW, Dodge PR: Unilateral pupillary dilatation during and immediately following seizures. *Neurol* 16:837–840, 1966.

27. Mitsumoto H: Ophthalmic aspects of subdural hematoma. *Cleveland Clinic Quarterly* 44(3):101, 1977.

28. Youmans J: Causes of shock with head injury. *J Trauma* 4:204, 1964.

29. Coats JB, Meirowsky A: *Neurological Surgery of Trauma.* Washington, DC, Office of the Surgeon General, Department of the Army, 1965, p 53.

30. Jones RK: Assessment of minimal head injuries: indications for in-hospital care. *Surg Neurol* 2:101, 1974.

31. Hull HF, Morrow G: Glucorrhea revisited. *JAMA* 234:1052, 1975.

32. Food and Drug Administration: Population Exposure to X-rays—U.S. 1970. Washington, D.C., Government Printing Office HEW Pub No. (FDA) 73-8047, November 1973.

33. Bell RS, Loop JW: The utility and futility of radiographic skull examinations for trauma. *N Engl J Med* 284:236–239, 1971.

34. Department of Health, Education and Welfare: Selection criteria reduce unnecessary skull x-rays. *FDA Drug Bulletin* 8(5):30 October-November 1978, p 30.

35. Eyes B et al: Post traumatic skull radiographs, time for a reappraisal. *Lancet* 2:85 July 1978.

36. Pilling H: *Proc R Soc Med* 69:755, 1976.

37. Rose J et al: Avoidable factors contributing to death after head injury. *Brit Med J* 2(6087):615, September 3, 1977.

38. Schwartz G et al: Trauma to the head, in *Principles and Practice of Emergency Medicine,* Philadelphia, WB Saunders Co, 1978 p. 607–627.

39. Goodman SJ, Cahan L, Chow AW: Subgaleal abscess. *West J Med* 127:169–172, August 1977.

40. James HE, Bruno LA, Schut L: Intracranial subarachnoid pressure monitoring in children. *Surg Neurol* 3:313, 1975.

41. Obrist WD, Thompson HK, Wang HS et al: Regional cerebral blood flow estimated by ^{133}Xenon inhalation. *Stroke* 6:245, 1975.

42. Bruce DA, Jennarelle TA, Langfitt, TW: Resuscitation from coma due to head injury. *Crit Care Med*

62

6(4):254–269, 1978.

43. Gennarelli TA, et al: Vascular and metabolic reactivity to changes in PCO_2 in head injured patients, in Bourke R (ed): *Proceedings of the Third Chicago Symposium in Neurological Trauma*, New York, Raven Press, 1978.

44. Ransohoff J: The effects of steroids on brain edema in man, in Reulen, HJ, Schurmann, K. (eds): *Steroids and Brain Edema*, New York, Springer-Verlag, 1972, p 211–218.

45. Gutterman P, Shenkin HA: Prognostic features in recovery from traumatic decerebration. *J Neurosurg* 32:330, 1970.

46. Faupel G, Reulen HS, Muller D, et al: Double blind study on the effects of steroids on severe closed head injury, in Pappus HM, Feindel W (eds): *Dynamics of Brain Edema*, New York, Springer-Verlag 1976, p 337–343.

47. Gobiet W, Bock WJ, Liesegang J, et al: Treatment of acute cerebral edema with high dose dexamethasone in Beks, J. WF, Bosch DA, Brock M (eds): *Intracranial Pressure III*. New York, Springer-Verlag 1976, p

231–235.

48. Feig PU, McCurdy DK: The hypertonic state. *N Engl J Med* 297:1444, 1977.

49. Goluboff B, Shenkin HA, Haft H: The effects of mannitol and urea on cerebral hemodynamics and cerebral spinal fluid pressure. *Neurol* 14:891–898, 1964.

50. Marshall LF, et al: Mannitol dose requirements in brain injured patients. *J Neurosurg* 48(2):169, February 1978.

51. Bourke R (ed): *Proceedings of the Third Chicago Symposium in Neurological Trauma*, New York, Raven Press, 1978.

52. Marshall LF, Shapiro MR: Barbiturate control of intracranial hypertension in head injury and other conditions, in Inguar DH, Lassen NA (eds): *Function, Metabolism, and Circulation*, Copenhagen, Munksgaard 1977, p 156–157.

53. Bruce DA, Schut L, Bruno LA, et al: Outcome following severe head injury in children. *J Neurosurg* 48:679, 1978.

Trauma of the Cervical Spine

James R. Roberts, M.D.
Assistant Professor in Emergency Medicine
The Medical College of Pennsylvania
Philadelphia, Pennsylvania

S ERIOUS CERVICAL SPINE injury occurs in 15 to 20% of patients with serious head injuries, but cervical spine injuries may not be as dramatic as head trauma and can be easily overlooked. Since spinal cord injury is so catastrophic, both psychologically and financially, its prevention and early detection are important priorities.

All too often a potentially reversible injury is converted into permanent neurological dysfunction because of simple human error. The prevention of needless tragedy is the goal of prehospital and emergency department care.

ETIOLOGY AND MECHANICS OF INJURY

The victims of spinal cord injuries are the young. Spinal cord injuries occur most commonly after a fall, in an automobile accident or during athletic activity, or as the result of penetrating trauma. Actual damage to the cord is the result of

64 complex flexion, extension, compressive or rotary forces transmitted through the spinal column.

Concussion, Contusion and Laceration of the Spinal Cord

Injuries to the cord are often associated with fracture or fracture-dislocation of the cervical spine, but massive injury may occur without readily identifiable signs of trauma from concussion, contusion or laceration of the spinal cord. Concussion of the spinal cord is a rather vague term used to describe a temporary loss of function, which is reversible in 24 to 48 hours. No neuropathological findings are consistently seen with spinal cord concussion, and it may be similar to cerebral concussion. The condition is quite rare.

Contusion of the cord is a bruise, associated with bleeding and necrosis and varying degrees of neurological deficit. The cord may undergo compression from heavy bleeding around the cord, a herniation of the intervertebral disc or a depressed fracture. Unlike the brain, the spinal cord tolerates compression very poorly for even short periods of time.

When the cord is actually torn or disrupted, the injury is termed a laceration. Although complete transection of the cord rarely occurs, in an anatomical sense, a physiologically complete transection is common. Contusion and laceration of the cord result in all degrees of disability ranging from minimal neurological deficit to complete loss of function. Injury to the spinal cord can also result from dislocation or rupture of the intravertebral discs. These injuries are not detected on routine x-rays and require myelography for definitive diagnosis.

Fractures

A variety of fracture patterns are seen with cervical spine injury.[1-3] Bursting or blowout fractures (a variant of the wedge compression fracture) are transmitted along the longitudinal axis of the vertebral bodies. Severe injury may occur with bursting fractures as the cord is injured by exploding bony fragments. Such an injury may result from hitting the head on a car roof. A specific bursting fracture involving the first cervical vertebra is termed Jefferson fracture. In general no cord damage occurs with a Jefferson fracture, possibly because the spinal canal is wide at the C_1 level.

When compressive forces are coupled with flexion or extension injuries, compression-wedge or tear-drop fractures may result. Fractures of the spinous processes are usually the result of pure extension forces. Linear fractures without displacement commonly involve transverse spinous processes or vertebral bodies, and unless they are unstable or involve the cord, these fractures rarely cause significant morbidity.

Of special note is the Hangman's fracture. Although this injury was originally described as a result of judicial hanging,[4] it may occur in automobile accidents and as a result of a suicide attempt. A Hangman's fracture is a bilateral fracture through the posterior neural arches of C_2 with or without dislocation of C_2 on C_3. The odontoid is not fractured. The mechanism is one of hyperextension, increased by the knot of the rope properly placed under the chin, and longitudinal traction, accentuated by weights around the ankles. Death is almost instantaneous if the hanging is performed properly.

Multiple fracture patterns are associated with diving injuries,[5] which occur frequently in younger patients and often result in permanent disability. The mechanism is one of hyperflexion producing fracture-dislocation. It is interesting that most diving injuries involving the cord are not associated with obvious head trauma, such as scalp lacerations or contusions. The precise mechanism of injury in diving accidents is unknown.

Many divers with cord injuries probably drown. Attempts to rescue swimmers from the water or to do cardiopulmonary resuscitation (CPR) by hyperextending the neck undoubtedly convert many incomplete injuries into complete paralysis.

Fracture-Dislocation

A simple nondisplaced fracture of the cervical spine is not catastrophic. Fracture-dislocation is, however, a most serious injury since the spinal cord is frequently involved. Fracture-dislocation of the cervical spine requires the expertise of an orthopedic surgeon and neurosurgeon, and should be treated with the utmost respect.

Fracture-dislocations may occur in any area, but often the upper and lower regions are commonly involved with relative sparing of the midportion of the spine. Ligamentous rupture and secondary bleeding can complicate the injury. Fracture-dislocations injuring the cord above C_5 are

often fatal due to respiratory arrest. Common sites of dislocations are C_1–C_2 (associated with odontoid fractures), C_2–C_3 (Hangman's fracture), C_5–C_6 and C_6–C_7 (falls, and diving and automobile accidents).

Cervical fracture-dislocation is usually, but not invariably, associated with direct head trauma.[6] Specifically, fracture-dislocation can occur when seat belts are worn in high-speed car accidents[7] and when hyperextension type injuries occur.

A unilateral rotary subluxation, not associated with a fracture, has been described.[3] It usually occurs in children without major trauma, probably from a hyperflexion-rotation mechanism. The patient presents without neurological deficit and appears to have torticollis. The diagnosis may be difficult to prove by x-ray, and usually the entity resolves without specific treatment or minimal manipulation. These injuries may be mistaken for simple neck sprains.

Whiplash

A sudden hyperextension of the spine with prolongation of the neck produces the well-known whiplash syndrome.[8,9] The neck is stretched by the force of the lower body moving forward, and by the backward and downward course of the head. Hyperextension produces the greatest injury since forward flexion is limited as the chin strikes the chest and lateral flexion is limited as the head hits the shoulders.

Whiplash injury is extremely common and is often seen by emergency medicine clinicians. It is common for this injury to develop 12 to 48 hours after an accident. It is frustrating for both patient and physician because no pathology can be detected in most cases yet the patient may have incapacitating pain. Patients often vaguely describe the whiplash yet describe the circumstances of the rear-end collision dramatically. Although there is an element of emotional or financial gain in legal cases involving whiplash injury, it has been found that successful litigation fails to relieve symptoms in almost half of the patients who have been followed for two years. Curiously, patients injured by flexion or lateral flexion injuries rarely institute lawsuits.

There is some anatomical basis for whiplash injury. A 15 mile-per-hour rear-end collision can accelerate the head with a force of 10G. Experimentally, sudden hyperextension results in a variety of soft-tissue injuries to the anterior neck muscles (sternocleidomastoid, scaleni and longus colli). These structures are damaged by tearing, stretching, microhemorrhage and edema. In addition, injury may involve the esophagus, trachea, longitudinal ligaments, intervertebral discs, nerve roots and vertebral artery. Most cases result in muscle or ligament sprain. Patients may complain of vague headache, neck and shoulder pain, lethargy, paresthesias, dizziness, vertigo or tinnitus.

Tinnitus is common and may be ascribed to vertebral artery spasm or cervical sympathetic irritation; however, the exact etiology is obscure. Dysphagia may result from pharyngeal edema or retropharyngeal hematoma in severe cases. Radicular pain does not necessarily indicate nerve root compression, and disc herniation associated with nerve root impingement is rare in these injuries. Paresthesias in the ulnar nerve distribution in the hand are felt to be the result of scalenus spasm. Mild, unrecognized cerebral contusion may accompany the cervical injury.[10]

Hyperextension injury in the presence of preexisting cervical pathology deserves special attention. It is well known that patients with cervical spondylosis, usually from osteoarthritis or ankylosing spondylitis,[11] are at greater risk following hyperextension injuries. With osteoarthritis the intervertebral foramina are narrowed and posterior osteophytes may be formed on the vertebral bodies. The spine is more rigid, and the bones are more brittle. Hyperextension allows the cord to be pinched between the bulging calcified ligamentum flavum and the posterior osteophytes causing nerve roots to be traumatized in a crowded foramina.

Spinal Shock

Spinal shock describes the immediate response of the spinal cord to injury. The neurological deficit may be reversible depending upon the specific pathology. Immediately following severe injury to the cord, there is a complete loss of all motor, sensory and reflex function distal to the site of injury, including loss of the Babinski and plantar reflexes and loss of vascular as well as muscular tone. Trauma does not always produce complete loss of function, and varying degrees of spinal shock may be seen, depending on the extent of cord damage. Without improvement of total spinal shock after 24 hours (and this improvement may be extremely subtle), the chance for any significant recovery is nil.

Total spinal shock results in a drop in blood pressure, often associated with a bradycardia—a point which may distinguish it from hypovolemic shock. There is immediate paralysis of the bladder and bowels, a sharp line of sensory loss and absence of sweating. A paralytic ileus develops, and occasionally there is priapism secondary to venous engorgement. A Horner's syndrome may be seen with lesions at the C_7–T_1 level.

If absolutely *no* motor, sensory or reflex activity is seen immediately following spinal cord injury, the chance for any significant recovery is minuscule. A phenomenon called sacral sparing cannot be overemphasized. The preservation of sacral segmental sensation and reflex is one of the most frequently overlooked neurological signs in patients with cervical cord injuries. The presence of sacral sparing indicates the spinal cord lesion is incomplete, and there is a significant chance of functional recovery. All efforts must be made to prevent any further injury if sacral sparing is noted.

DIAGNOSIS OF CERVICAL SPINE INJURY

Any unconscious or traumatized patient should be diagnosed with "possible cervical spine injury" until proven otherwise. On rare occasions, a conscious patient with multiple trauma may have a serious cervical spine injury without neurological deficit or neck pain.[12] At great risk are patients with serious head trauma. In the emergency department, the lateral cervical spine x-ray is far more important than the skull x-ray in diagnosing cervical cord injury.

The Examination

Complete paralysis makes the diagnosis of cervical cord injury easy. Subtle findings, especially in the unconscious patient, should also alert the physician to serious injury. For example, the finding of seat belt ecchymosis in an unconscious patient raises the possibility of a neck injury.

VITAL SIGNS

Following severe spinal cord injury, the blood pressure is often reduced due to loss of vasomotor control. Although hypovolemia may also be present, spinal shock produces a different type of hypotension, which may be distinguished from true hypovolemia.[13] In uncomplicated spinal shock, the pulse is slow and strong. The patient is usually oriented and alert, and the skin is warm and dry. Spinal shock hypotension responds poorly to volume replacement but may respond well to neosynephrine infusion.[14] The hypotension may persist for weeks or months and occasionally is permanent.

If the cord injury is proximal to or involves the origin of the phrenic nerve (C_3, C_4, C_5), respiration is impossible, and patients usually die immediately. If the lesion is below C_5 and above the origin of the intercostal nerves from the thoracic cord, evidence of diaphragmatic breathing is seen. An unconscious patient who has no intercostal movement but does have abdominal breathing should be considered to have cord transection below C_5.

68 Hypothermia may be associated with spinal cord injury, due to a loss of thermoregulatory mechanisms mediated by the spinal cord. Spinal cord injuries may go unnoticed in patients suffering from extreme hypothermia.[15] The cord injury itself may precipitate profound hypothermia, especially if the patient is exposed to low ambient temperature.[16]

Physical Examination

A distended bladder, gastric dilatation and paralytic ileus are seen with spinal cord injuries. Aspiration is always a threat, so early nasogastric (NG) suction is in order before vomiting takes place. Further cord damage by vomiting or neck motion during passage of the NG tube must be avoided. Incontinence, due to overflow of a distended bladder or colon, may signal neurological impairment in a patient without obvious spinal injury. A distended abdomen and loss of peristalsis may not only signal spinal shock, but may also indicate a surgical intra-abdominal injury.

Because sensory input is disrupted, the patient will not experience pain from a ruptured liver or spleen, ectopic pregnancy, appendicitis, peritonitis or the like. Failure to diagnose a perforated bladder in a paralyzed trauma patient may lead to early death from sepsis. Priapism is infrequently encountered but is diagnostic.

NEUROLOGICAL EXAMINATION

Neurological changes may be grouped into the following categories, each of which requires careful examination: voluntary muscle power, sensibility, reflex activity and sphincter control.

Sensory Examination. Sensory modalities provide a great deal of information in localizing spinal cord lesions. Subtle changes in sensation are picked up by careful attention to details. The entire sensory examination cannot be done with only a safety pin; pricking the skin with a pin can be the last sensory modality to be lost at a given level. Painful sensation, as seen with a pin prick and the appreciation of temperature, travels in the lateral spinal-thalamic tract, which carries impulses up the opposite side of the cord from the origin of the lesion.

The posterior columns carry the fibers for the sensation of position and movement (such as the up or down position of the big toe), the fibers for two-point discrimination, vibratory sensation (from, for example, a tuning fork) and the sensation of pressure. These fibers transmit impulses on the same side as the origin of the impulse.

Light touch, e.g., stroking the skin with a cotton swab, travels in the anterior spinothalamic tracts, although the sensory modality of the tracts has limited clinical value in localizing injuries to the spinal cord.

In cases of cord transection, all sensation distal to the lesion is completely lost. One can obtain a reasonable approximation of the level of the spinal cord injury by demonstrating loss of sensation to pin scratch, in the area of specific sensory dermatomes.[17] (See Figure 1.) The initial examination should test sensation in the lateral forearm (C_5), the thumb (C_6), the index finger (C_7), the little finger (C_8) and the medial forearm (T_1).

FIGURE 1. SENSORY DERMATOMES OF THE UPPER AND LOWER LIMBS

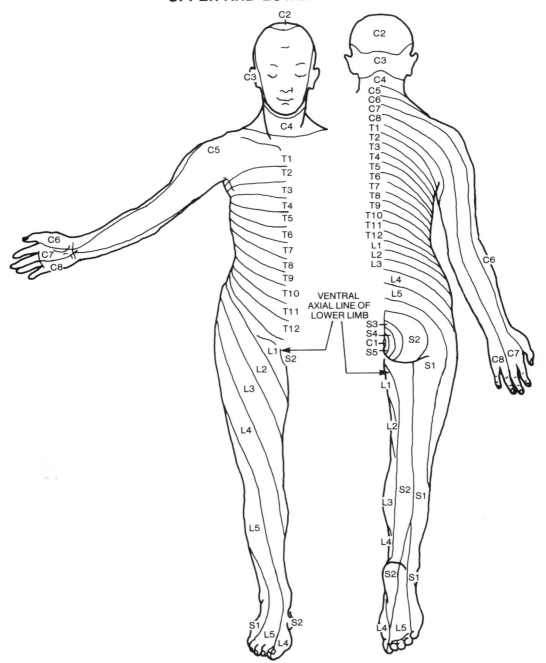

70

The Concept of Sacral Sparing. Sensory tracts of the sacral segments are located in the periphery of the cords in the sensory columns. They are likely to escape injury from lesions, such as the central cord syndrome, which produce hemorrhage or necrosis within the cord substance. Therefore the sensory examination must include investigation of this important area, for any sign of sacral sparing immediately following cord injury indicates that the lesion is *incomplete*. A relatively hopeless situation may be differentiated from a potentially reversible lesion.

The sacral examination should include an evaluation of not only sphincter tone, but also of the perianal skin sensation (anal wink reflex of the sphincter following pin prick) and of the bulbocavernosus reflex (squeezing of the penis or vulva, or pulling on a Foley catheter causing sphincter contraction). Although the absence of sacral sparing during spinal shock does not always preclude recovery, its presence is a hopeful prognostic sign. Certainly its presence should prompt meticulous attention to prevention of further neurological injury.

Reflex Evaluation. During spinal shock all deep tendon reflexes below the site of injury, including pathological reflexes such as the Babinski reflex, are absent. Plantar responses may return in a few hours as flexor responses. With minimal reflex testing, the level of spinal cord injury may be approximated. Complete paralysis of all limbs indicates a lesion at C_5 or above. The deltoids are innervated at C_5 (shoulder shrug) and the biceps and triceps at C_6 (occasionally the biceps reflex may be retained in the absence of triceps

reflex indicating a C_5–C_6 lesion), and squeezing of the hands is dependent on an intact C_7. Spreading of the fingers is mediated by C_8–T_1. There is some degree of overlapping in cervical segment reflex testing. On the basis of careful physical and neurological examination including sensory examination, especially for sacral sparing, and evaluation of the reflexes, a number of specific syndromes of spinal cord injuries can be identified as outlined below.[13,17,18]

Brown-Sequard Syndrome

Brown-Sequard syndrome is hemitransection of the cord, and it usually follows knife or missile injuries or unilateral articular process fractures. The syndrome consists of ipsilateral motor paralysis (corticospinal tract), loss of position and vibratory sense (posterior column) and contralateral loss of pain and temperature sensation (lateral spinalthalamic tract).

Central Cord Syndrome

The central cord syndrome results from microhemorrhage, edema and vascular insufficiency of the central gray matter of the cord. The lateral corticospinal tracts are especially vulnerable. Because the upper corticospinal tracts are nearer the center of the cord, there is disproportionate weakness of the upper extremities when compared to the lower extremities. There may be bilateral loss of pain and temperature sensation, and if the lesion is particularly widespread, position and vibratory sense are impaired. There is varying involvement of the bladder.

The mechanism of this syndrome is

variable but the usual cause is hypertension. This is particularly seen in patients with cervical spondylosis and posterior osteophyte formation. This lesion commonly does not involve a fracture of the bony spine.

Anterior Cord Syndrome

Anterior cord syndrome results from cervical compression and hyperflexion injuring the anterior spinal cord or the anterior spinal artery. Motor paralysis of the upper and lower limbs with loss of pain and temperature sensation bilaterally are noted. The dorsal columns are spared, and position and vibratory sense are preserved.

Radiological Examination

Although complete, irreversible paralysis is possible without demonstrable x-ray findings, and although it is difficult to relate radiographical signs with neurological function, all patients with neck trauma should have x-rays of the cervical spine.[19-21] The most frequent error is to accept an incomplete study, especially by omitting the odontoid open mouth view and failing to obtain views of the C_7-T_1 area. Since most of the injuries involve the proximal and distal areas of the spine, it is imperative to obtain all views. Various techniques such as the swimmer's view for C_7 are available and should be utilized.

Three people are needed to obtain adequate x-rays of the traumatized neck—one to hold the head, the second to put downward traction on the arms and the third to take the x-ray. The *portable* lateral cervical spine film is the first x-ray to be taken in cases of multiple trauma. If the patient must go to the x-ray department, the physician in charge should be in attendance. A full series should be obtained, but flexion-extension views are extremely dangerous in the acute situation because motion of the head to obtain these views may damage the cord in an unstable injury. Old fractures may be differentiated from new ones by use of a bone scan.

Although alignment of the cervical spine should always be noted, other factors are important. (See Figure 2.) X-ray evaluation of the soft tissues of the neck is necessary to analyze fully the cervical spine. Whiplash injuries may manifest reversal of cervical lordosis and straightening of the curve of the spine, signifying muscle spasm. Straightening of the spine can be mimicked by assuming a military position with the chin tightly tucked on the neck. Straightening of the spine on lateral neck x-ray may be overrated as a sign of injury.

The width of the prevertebral soft tissue space between the anterior border of the body of C_3 and the posterior border of the air column in the hypopharynx should not exceed 5 mm in the adult. Widening of this space indicates hemorrhage, pushing the air column forward. This rule does not hold true for areas below C_4 because the esophagus is transposed between the trachea and the spine making strict adherence to a measurement quite difficult. Air in the prevertebral space is a sign of rupture of the trachea, esophagus or pneumomediastinum, or a sign of a pneumothorax.

Children present a slightly more com-

FIGURE 2. NORMAL LATERAL CERVICAL SPINE

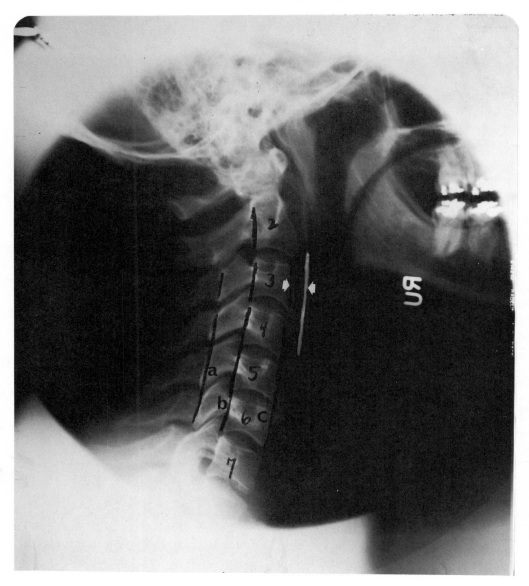

Although a full cervical spine series is needed for accurate evaluation, the lateral C-Spine x-ray has a wealth of information and may be the only view available in an emergency. Alignment is judged by a line connecting the following structures: (a) the inner cortical margin of the spinous processes (b) the posterior portion of the vertebral bodies and (c) the anterior portion of the vertebral bodies. Each line should form a smooth, continuous curve, and disruption of the curve may indicate fracture or dislocation.

The prevertebral soft-tissue space (between arrows) is best measured between the posterior border of the pharyngeal air column and the anterior border of C_3 or C_4. This space should not exceed 5 mm in an adult or about 1/3 rd of the width of C_4. The space is normally a few millimeters wider in children, especially during expiration. Widening of the space suggests edema or bleeding.

plex problem in radiographical examination. The prevertebral tissue may buckle and simulate a mass lesion unless the film is taken during peak inspiration and in extension. In addition, children have hypermobile spines, and an apparent subluxation of C_2 on C_3 may be suspected unless one carefully measures the posterior cervical line.[19]

The odontoid process is often difficult to evaluate radiographically. It may be seen on the lateral film or on an open mouth view. The odontoid process usually fractures at its base. On the lateral view, the distance between the anterior portion of the odontoid process and the posterior portion of the anterior arch of C_1 should not exceed 2 to 4 mm. (See Figure 3.) There are congenital anomalies of the odontoid which may mimic fractures, especially nonunion of the odontoid with the body of C_2.

One may obtain an idea of stability of cervical fractures by radiographical examination.[2,21,22] If a vertebral body is displaced anteriorly over the underlying body on the lateral film, it is a *stable* fracture. This indicates unilateral dislocation of one interfacetal joint with rupture of the interspinous ligament at that level but an intact annulus and posterior intervertebral ligament.

If the anterior dislocation is greater than one half of the width of the vertebral body it is an *unstable* fracture. This indicates bilateral dislocation of the intervertebral joints, and rupture of the annulus and posterior ligaments. Obviously, the above is an approximation which should be viewed cautiously.

TREATMENT

The goals of emergency department treatment are two-fold: (1) the diagnosis must be suspected and confirmed, and (2) further injury must be prevented. Treatment begins at the scene of the accident. All patients should be checked for gross neurological dysfunction, and the spine should be gently palpated *before* the patient is moved. The lack of physical findings or absence of pain should not deter specific precautions concerning neck injuries.

Moving and Positioning. A spine board or cervical collar should be applied before the patient is extricated from a vehicle. Crash helmets or football helmets should not be removed outside of the hospital. Patients should be moved as if they were logs, and the emergency medicine clinician in charge should stand at the head of the patient and be responsible for protecting the neck during moving. The head should be in a neutral position without flexion or extension, and slight longitudinal traction should be maintained during transfer.

Under no circumstance should the patient sit or stand. The neck should be stabilized with sandbags, towels, cervical collars or a vacuum bean-bag type apparatus until traction can be applied. The patient should be placed on a hard, flat surface, and no pillow is used. If at all possible, the patient should be moved on a stryker frame or other lifting device. There is a possibility of aspiration with any patient lying supine especially with associated head trauma that predisposes to vomiting. Specific care should be taken to protect the necks of patients injured in

FIGURE 3.   ODONTOID VIEWS

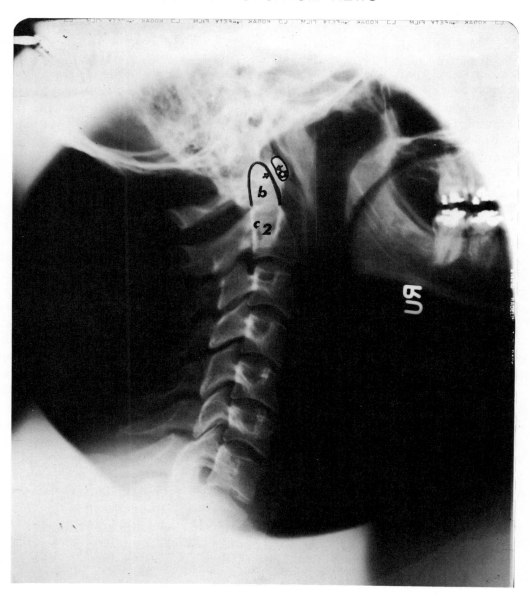

An open mouth view of the odontoid process should always be ordered, but it may be difficult to obtain in some patients. Although tomograms are often needed for definite diagnosis, this lateral view is often helpful. The important area to evaluate is the prevertebral space (between arrows). This is the area between (a) the posterior margin of the anterior arch of C_1, the atlas, and (b) the anterior surface of the odontoid process. If this space exceeds 4 mm in an adult on the lateral film, a fracture of the base of the odontoid must be suspected.

diving accidents, since the injury is often unexpected.

Airway and Breathing. Maintaining an airway is particularly difficult in patients with spinal injury because most methods for providing an airway are associated with motion of the head. However, esophageal obturator airway can be used both in the field and in the emergency department.

Intubation over a fiberoptic bronchoscope is ideal. Tracheal intubation via the "blind" nasotracheal route is quite acceptable. If the endotracheal route is the only possible method, it may be attempted by having an assistant stabilize the neck and perform a jaw thrust maneuver while the physician performs the intubation. If air exchange is judged adequate and there is no problem with secretions, the patient should not be intubated until x-rays are obtained.

Hypotension. The hypotension of spinal shock does not usually require aggressive treatment. The military anti-shock trouser (MAST) suit or simple elevation of the legs is usually sufficient. If shock is severe, neosynephrine can be used as a pressor agent. Causes for hypovolemia should be sought.

Traction. Unfortunately, most mistakes which result in worsening of the cervical trauma occur before the patient reaches the hospital. This is often done by well-meaning people who are in a hurry to "help" the patient. It is estimated that one out of ten patients experience an increase in cord damage during the period of immediate care.[1]

Once the patient reaches the hospital, cervical traction should be immediately applied if there is any indication of serious cervical injury. This may be done before

FIGURE 4.   HALTER TRACTION

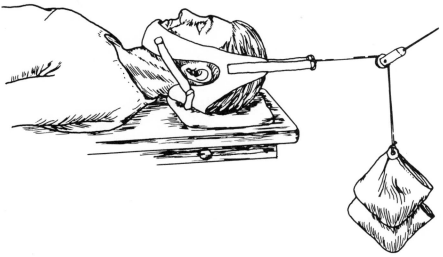

Halter traction may be applied before x-rays are taken. The direction of pull must be in line with the vertebral column.

76

x-rays are obtained. The best way to apply emergency traction is by use of a halter strap with 10 to 15 pounds of traction.[22] (See Figure 4.) Skeletal traction is best left to the neurosurgeon or orthopedic surgeon.

Adjunctive Techniques. A Foley catheter is indicated early in the care of spinal injuries to avoid overdistension and stasis of the bladder. A nasogastric (NG) tube should be passed in the emergency department to avoid the hazards of gastric dilation and aspiration. One must be careful when passing the tube to avoid further injury to the cord.

High-dose antibiotics which cross the blood-brain barrier, such as penicillin, ampicillin, or chloramphenicol should be used if a penetrating injury is present.

Corticosteroids. Although there is no actual evidence that steroids will reduce morbidity in spinal cord injuries, they are routinely given early in the emergency department protocol.[14] Dexamethasone, 10 mg IV initially, followed by 4 mg every four hours, is a reasonable choice.

Whiplash Injury. Soft-tissue injury to the neck is particularly troublesome to treat and slow to resolve. Treatment is empirical at best. Mild injuries are treated with aspirin, local heat and rest. Muscle relaxants are probably of some value, perhaps for their sedating qualities which promote rest. Rest, taking the weight of the head off the neck, is particularly important and often underemphasized. More severe injuries may need complete bed rest, cervical traction and narcotics for pain relief, although narcotics should be used sparingly. Local injection of steroids and lido-

caine is indicated if there is point tenderness or trigger spots are identified. Ultrasound and modalities of heat application can often be of significant value, and refractory cases can be referred to the physical therapy department.

Cervical collars should not be given in mild cases, but if they are used they should be worn 24 hours a day, especially at night, and a pillow should be avoided. If pain persists for more than two weeks, reasonable results have been obtained with the short-term (seven to ten days) use of potent anti-inflammatory agents, such as the combination of phenylbutazone and prednisone (Sterazolidin®), or others (Butazolidin® or Indocin®) if no contraindication exists.

Possible Advances in Therapy. Local hypothermic perfusion[23] and hyperbaric oxygen therapy[24] have been suggested for severe injuries, but beneficial results are unproven. There is some evidence that catecholamines may migrate to the area of spinal cord injury causing injury by local vasomotor changes that may be prevented by alphamethyl-tyrosine, but again clinical trials are lacking.[25]

SUMMARY

Since trauma to the cervical spine may have devastating consequences, the neck must be given high priority in all multiply injured patients. A careful and rapid physical examination and high index of suspicion for cervical spinal cord injury may prevent a stable injury from iatrogenically becoming a major catastrophe. The subtleties of a neurological examination, complexities of spinal cord physiology and the intricacies of the radiological examination must all be in the armamentarium of the emergency medicine clinician to assure a successful outcome in patients with serious neck injuries.

REFERENCES

1. Rogers W, Forsythe: Fractures and dislocations of the cervical spine. *J Bone Joint Surg* 39:321, 1957.
2. Beatson TR: Fractures and dislocations of the cervical spine. *J Bone Joint Surg* 45B:21–35, 1963.
3. DePalma AF: *The Management of Fractures and Dislocations* ed 2. Philadelphia, WB Saunders Co, 1970.
4. Wood-Jones F: The ideal lesion produced by judicial hanging. *Lancet,* 1913, p 53.
5. Kewalramani LS, Orth MD, Taylor RG: Injuries to the cervical spine from diving accidents. *J Trauma* 15(2):130–141, 1975.
6. Huelke AF, Mendelsohn RA, States JD, et al. Cervical fracture and fracture dislocations sustained without head impact. *J Trauma* 18:533–538, 1978.
7. Taylor TK, Nade S, Bannister JH: Seat belt fractures of the cervical spine. *J Bone Joint Surg* 58:328–331, 1976.
8. Macnab I: Acceleration injuries of the cervical spine. *J Bone Joint Surg* 46A:1779–1799, 1964.
9. Gay JR, Abbott KH: Common whiplash injuries of the neck. *JAMA* 152:1698–1704, 1953.
10. Ommaya AK, Fass F, Yarnell P: Whiplash injury and brain damage. *JAMA* 204:285–289, 1968.
11. Osgood CP, Abbasyn M, Mathews T: Multiple spine fracture in ankylosing spondylitis. *J Trauma* 15(2):163, 1975.
12. Maull KI, Sachatello CR: Avoiding a pitfall in resuscitation: the painless cervical fractures. *South Med J* 70(4):477–478, 1977.
13. Hardy AG, Rossier AB: *Spinal Cord Injuries: Orthopedic and Neurological Aspects,* thieme ed. Publishing Sciences Group, Inc, 1975.
14. Schwartz G, et al: Spinal injuries, in *Principles and Practice of Emergency Medicine.* Philadelphia, WB Saunders Co, 1978 pp 618–627.
15. Truscott DG, Firor WB, Clein LJ: Accidental profound hypothermia. *Arch Surg* 106(2):216–218, 1973.
16. Bova CM: Accidental hypothermia precipitated by spinal cord lesions. *JACEP* in press.
17. Grant JCB: *An Atlas of Anatomy,* ed 5. Baltimore, Williams & Wilkins Co, 1962.
18. Marrar C: The pattern of neurological damage as an aid to the diagnosis of the mechanism in cervical spine injuries. *J Bone Joint Surg* 56A:1648, 1974.
19. Harris JH, Harris WH: *The Radiology of Emergency Medicine.* Baltimore, Williams & Wilkins Co, 1975.
20. King DM: Fractures and dislocation of the cervical spine. *J Bone Joint Surg* 45:21, 1963.
21. Whitley JE, Forsyth HF: The classification of cervical spine injuries. *Am J Roentgenol Radium Ther Nucl Med* 83:633, 1960.
22. The Committee on Trauma American College of Surgeons: *Early Care of the Injured Patient.* Philadelphia, WB Saunders Co, 1976.
23. Albin MS, White RJ, Acosta-Roa G, et al: Study of functional recovery produced by delayed localizing cooling after spinal cord injury in primates. *J Neurosurg* 29:113, 1968.
24. Kelly OL, Lassiter KRL, Vongsvivut A, et al: Effects of hyperbasic oxygenation and tissue oxygen studies in experimental paraplegia. *J Neurosurg* 36:425–429, 1972.
25. Osterholm JL, Matthews GL: Altered norepinephrine metabolism following experimental spinal cord injury. *J Neurosurg* 36:395–401, 1972.

Management of Chest Injuries

Martin S. Kohn, M.D.
Department of Emergency Medicine
Good Samaritan Hospital
San Jose, California

INJURIES of the chest are a common problem in the emergency department. In this era of high-speed vehicle transportation, chest injury is the major contributor to death in 25% of accidents and a factor in 25 to 50% of the remainder.[1] Violent crime and nonautomotive accidents also contribute to an increasing occurrence of chest trauma.[2]

Effective management of chest injuries depends on reversing conditions that prevent normal physiological function of organs. Each specific injury to the thoracic cage and its contents will exert some particular restriction on the ability of the heart to pump blood or the lungs to exchange air and oxygenate blood. By understanding the pathophysiological mechanisms of chest injury and how to counteract them, emergency medicine clinicians can save lives. Clearing the airway or judicious use of a hollow needle can tame a life-threatening injury in seconds. The opportunity to reverse an otherwise fatal course makes the manage-

80 ment of chest trauma both compelling and satisfying.

Basic principles of evaluation and management of chest injury must be followed regardless of the precise injury. As with any emergency situation, a rapid but comprehensive evaluation of the airway, breathing and circulation is mandatory. Appropriate general resuscitative measures should be instituted. Many patients have multiple injuries. The signs and symptoms of these injuries often overlap each other, so the diagnosis may be obscured by associated injuries. A further peril is that the most lethal injury may, initially, be the least apparent. The examiner must respond to obvious injuries, but not so hastily that the possibility of other problems is ignored. In one series, 66% of patients with serious chest trauma had major extrathoracic injuries.[3]

Several categories of symptoms and signs are most relevant to the evaluation of chest trauma. Respiratory distress is the most common sign.[4] The distress may reflect cardiovascular, pulmonary or chest wall injury and may present as pain with respiration, shortness of breath or simply tachypnea. Cyanosis signifies severe cardiopulmonary compromise.

Mechanical, or musculoskeletal, abnormalities of the chest may give clues to the source of respiratory distress. External evidence of injury, such as ecchymoses, abrasions or lacerations, suggests locations of internal injuries. Unequal motion of the two sides of the thorax or paradoxical motion of a portion of the chest help localize the site of ventilatory abnormalities. Subcutaneous emphysema reflects air leakage from the pulmonary tree or esophagus.[4]

Breath sounds, normally an important part of any physical examination, may be deceptive in evaluating chest trauma. Markedly diminished breath sounds may indicate a collapsed lung or merely splinting from a chest wall contusion. At the same time, normal breath sounds do not preclude serious pathology, such as collapse of a lung.

Cardiac examination should initially include auscultation for muffled or irregular heart sounds, murmurs or clicks. Displacement of the apical impulse may indicate shifting of the thoracic contents. Peripheral pulses and blood pressures should be checked as indicators of vascular integrity.

Essentially there are 12 categories of chest trauma; six require urgent attention in both the field and emergency department. Pneumothorax, particularly tension pneumothorax, hemothorax, flail chest, pericardial tamponade, penetrating heart wounds and airway obstruction require prompt intervention in the field. Myocardial or pulmonary contusion and rupture of the esophagus, aorta, diaphragm or mainstem bronchus are life-threatening problems, but usually require diagnostic and supportive care rather than definitive treatment in the field or emergency department.

PNEUMOTHORAX

Pneumothorax is a consequence of either blunt or penetrating injury to the lung, tracheobronchial tree or esophagus, with leakage of air into the pleural space. It is usually associated with shortness of breath and often with pleuritic pain. The term simple pneumothorax means that the lung is prevented from expanding due to air in the ipsilateral pleural space, without other complication. An open pneumothorax describes air in the pleural space and an open wound in the chest wall through which air flows during attempts at respiration. Tension pneumothorax occurs when air accumulates in the pleural space at a sufficient rate to compress both the ipsilateral and contralateral lungs as well as the mediastinal structures. Tension pneumothorax produces both hemodynamic and respiratory compromise, and is the most dangerous type of pneumothorax.

The objective of treatment for pneumothorax is to reexpand the lung to restore as near normal ventilation as possible. High-flow oxygen should be administered first. If the patient is relatively stable, there is time to initiate supportive treatment and confirm the diagnosis with a chest x-ray. The radiograph most often shows a partial pneumothorax, with the edge of the partially expanded lung bordering an area with normal lung markings and an area of air density with no vascular markings (the intrapleural air).[5] If no pneumothorax is seen, another film taken during the expiratory phase of respiration may be helpful. During expiration, the relative size of the air volume trapped in the pleural space increases relative to that of the lung, and a small pneumothorax may be more easily seen.

A patient with a simple pneumothorax involving more than 15% of the lung area should be treated with a chest tube to reexpand the lung.[6] The tube should be inserted in the fourth or fifth intercostal space, in the mid-axillary line, on the affected side. Bilateral pneumothorax requires bilateral chest tubes. After adequate skin preparation and local anesthesia, a 3 to 5 cm incision should be made down to the level of the intercostal muscles, but no deeper. A blunt instrument, such as a hemostat or Kelly clamp, should be used to complete the entry into the pleural cavity. The entrance hole through the pleura should be over the upper edge of the rib to avoid intercostal nerves and vessels. Penetration of the pleural space is indicated by air rushing through the incision. The tract should be kept open with the blunt instrument while the tube is inserted. A large Pean clamp, closed over the distal end of the tube during insertion, permits direction of the tube through the tract, and posteriorly and superiorly into the pleural cavity. (See Figure 1.) The tube should be inserted far enough so that the distal drainage holes are not exposed. If there is only air, and no fluid, in the pleural space, a relatively small tube, such as a No. 24, is adequate. If blood is present, then a larger tube, such as a No. 36, is used. The wound should be closed with silk suture. Gauze sponges, either dry or petrolatum impregnated, should be placed around the catheter site, and the catheter well secured with tape to prevent motion and pain. The chest tube is then connected to constant suction through a water seal, equivalent to 15 to 20 cm of water. Most commonly, complete

82

FIGURE 1. CLAMP USED TO HOLD AND DIRECT CHEST TUBE

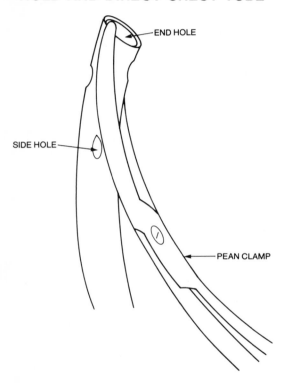

END HOLE

SIDE HOLE

PEAN CLAMP

reexpansion of the lung is seen on follow-up x-ray.

If the patient has an open, or sucking, chest wound complicating the pneumothorax, the wound should be covered but not sealed. Sealing the wound may cause a tension pneumothorax. Once a chest tube has been inserted, the wound may then be sealed with petrolatum gauze without a tension pneumothorax developing.

If the respiratory condition of a patient deteriorates progressively, then a tension pneumothorax must be suspected. Distended neck veins, distension of the injured side of the chest and displacement of the cardiac impulse away from the injured side add to the suspicion.[6] If there is time, insertion of a chest tube relieves tension and reverses deterioration. If the patient declines too rapidly or is not yet in the hospital, then a large needle, 15 or 16 gauge, should be inserted into the chest, over the top of the fifth rib in the anterior axillary line. If a tension pneumothorax is present, there will be a rush of exiting air and a dramatic relief of symptoms. If the situation does not improve, the procedure should be repeated on the other side of the chest. Once the tension pneumothorax is relieved, a chest tube is inserted, even prior to obtaining a chest x-ray, as any delay may allow the pneumothorax to redevelop.

HEMOTHORAX

Hemothorax is the accumulation of blood in the pleural space. The blood may be present alone, or in combination with air as a hemopneumothorax. Hemothorax is suspected when, in addition to the signs and symptoms of pneumothorax, indications of fluid in the chest, such as dullness to percussion, are noted. Blood in the pleural space may have all the adverse effects of air in the pleural space, plus the additional problem of hypovolemia if the blood accumulation is sufficient.

Blood in the pleural space will generally remain fluid, at least for the time course of emergency care. Thus hemothorax can best be demonstrated as a fluid level seen on an upright chest film.[5] A radiograph taken in the supine position only shows a generalized increase in density on the affected side. A lateral decubitus film may show the hemothorax if the patient cannot be moved to the erect position. If the chest radiograph demonstrates a straight interface between the pleural fluid and the lung density above it, with no meniscus, then a pneumothorax exists, even if none can be seen.

Field treatment consists of oxygen and a large-bore catheter for fluid replacement. In the emergency department, a large diameter chest tube should be inserted with the same technique as described for pneumothorax. Reexpansion of the lung is often the only treatment needed to control the bleeding that produced the hemothorax. The initial volume of blood removed by the chest tube should be recorded. An initial loss of 1000 cc has a high correlation with subsequent need for thoracotomy in the operating room.[7,8] The amount of continuing drainage should be recorded. Continued blood loss of 500 cc per hour is an indication for thoracotomy.[2, 7–9]

Extremely active bleeding, indicating that the patient cannot be supported by intravenous solutions and blood to survive for surgery in the operating room, justifies thoracotomy in the emergency department. Such a procedure is undertaken in the hope that the source of bleeding can be easily identified and clamped to help stabilize the patient.

In institutions with the equipment to perform autotransfusion, blood collected in a sterile fashion from the thoracostomy tube is well suited for autotransfusion. Until recently, this procedure was limited to university medical centers and larger municipal hospitals. However, the necessary equipment can now be found in some community hospitals.[10]

AIRWAY OBSTRUCTION

Obstruction of the airway can be due to foreign body, blood, vomitus or injury to the tracheobronchial tree itself. Material in the upper airway can be removed manually under direct vision. Blood or vomitus in the lower trachea and upper bronchi can be cleared with suction after the airway has been controlled with an endotracheal or nasotracheal tube. Foreign bodies may require bronchoscopy for removal.

PULMONARY CONTUSION AND FLAIL CHEST

Pulmonary contusion is usually the result of blunt trauma to the lung. It is characterized by edema and blood in the alveolae and interstitium. The contusion typically appears on the chest radiograph as a patchy or homogenous infiltrate with a nonsegmental distribution.

Fracture of three or more adjacent ribs, each in more than one place, can produce an unstable area of the chest wall, or flail chest.[11] This flail segment will not actively participate in respiratory effort. It may, in fact, move paradoxically, that is, inward with inspiration and outward with expiration.

Initial management in the field consists of external stabilization of the flail segment either with the hands, with a soft weighted object such as sand bags or by rolling the patient on the affected side to splint the flail segment.[11] In the emergency department, the flail segment should be similarly stabilized while the injury is being evaluated.

It has been traditionally stated that the

84

paradoxical motion of the flail segment is the major cause of the respiratory compromise.[11,12] There is now some strong evidence that a major cause of the respiratory compromise ascribed to flail chest is, indeed, a consequence of the underlying pulmonary contusion. Trinkle has noted that patients with other conditions that cause paradoxical motion, such as a paralyzed diaphragm or after pectus excavatum repair, do not require mechanical ventilation.[12] He argues that lung abnormalities associated with flail chest actually cause the respiratory compromise, not the paradoxical movement per se. In addition, animal studies indicate that pulmonary contusion is increased by overhydration, particularly with crystalloid.[13] The contusion is reduced in size if fluids are restricted.

Based on these two ideas, Trinkle's regimen included:

- restriction of fluids to 1000 cc at resuscitation and 50 cc per hour thereafter;
- intravenous methylprednisolone, 500 mg, every six hours for three days;
- plasma, 50 cc per hour;
- replacement of blood loss by either whole blood or plasma;
- vigorous pulmonary toilet;
- pain control with intercostal nerve blocks and narcotics;
- oxygen by mask to keep arterial PO_2 above 60 mm Hg.

Endotracheal intubation and mechanical ventilation was reserved for those patients whose PO_2 fell below 60 mm Hg.

In a series of 30 patients, the group treated with Trinkle's regimen had higher survival rates, fewer complications and shorter hospitalizations than did patients with comparable injuries receiving the more classical treatment with prolonged positive pressure ventilation. In a subsequent group of 50 patients, 25 needed a brief period of mechanical ventilation, but only five required more than ten days on the respirator. The value of management oriented toward the pulmonary contusion has been confirmed by Shackford et al.[14] They emphasize the importance of pain control in improving respiration, and the decrease in infections and tracheal stenosis with the more selective regimen.

Many clinicians advocate positive pressure ventilation to counteract the flail chest until the fractures stabilize; others prefer mechanical stabilization of the fractures with struts, staples, clips and wires. The existence of several popular approaches to one disease usually means that no single approach is always appropriate. The relative contribution of pulmonary contusion and paradoxical chest wall motion to respiratory distress may vary according to the patient.

However, it is clear that many patients suffering from flail chest can be treated conservatively. Therefore, the emergency medicine clinician must stabilize the patient in a manner that does not complicate later treatment.

A flail chest victim, with adequate respiration (PO_2 greater than 60 mm Hg on room air) and blood pressure, needs only supplemental oxygen, analgesia and careful fluid restoration. A patient with an extensive chest wall injury, poor respiratory effort and hypovolemia from associated injuries requires endotracheal intubation and aggressive volume replacement. Reasoned, but aggressive, treatment in the emergency department is in the patient's best interest. If the initial inclination is to intubate the patient, then it is appropriate to do so. If at a later time the patient does not require active airway control, the tube can be removed. The consequences of not intubating a patient who needs controlled ventilation far outweigh the risks of intubating a patient who would have survived without it.

Similarly, excess crystalloid may extend the area of contusion, so the volume of fluid given to the patient should be restricted. Should the patient be hypotensive from hypovolemia, of course, the hypovolemia takes precedence. One should have the same concern for overhydration of the patient with pulmonary contusion as for the patient with a history of congestive heart failure.

PERICARDIAL TAMPONADE

Either blunt or penetrating injury can precipitate the accumulation of blood in the pericardial sac. If a sufficiently large volume of blood occupies the sac, then cardiac filling, and consequently cardiac output, is reduced.[15] Signs and symptoms suggestive of pericardial tamponade include hypotension, tachycardia, respiratory distress, distended neck veins (or elevated central venous pressure) and muffled heart sounds. Pulsus paradoxus, a drop in the systolic blood pressure of more than 10 mm Hg between expiration and inspiration, is also characteristic of pericardial tamponade.[6] However, the absence of any of the signs or symptoms does not preclude significant tamponade.

A mild tamponade may respond to a fluid challenge. The increase in venous filling pressure can improve cardiac filling to produce a modest increase in cardiac output. A transient improvement at best, such an increase should not delay more definitive therapy. Pericardiocentesis, the draining of fluid from the pericardial sac, is the mainstay of emergency therapy for tamponade.

Ideally, the anterior chest and upper abdomen should be prepared with an antiseptic. A three-inch, 18-gauge spinal or cardiac needle, with a metal hub, attached to a 35 or 50 cc syringe, should be inserted in the right paraxiphoid space. The needle should then be aimed toward the left shoulder, at an angle of about 35° with the skin surface. From this point on, electrocardiographic monitoring is helpful. The electrocardiographic apparatus should be set up to record a typical chest lead, but the exploring electrode should be attached, using a wire with an alligator clip at each end, to the hub of the needle. As the syringe and needle are advanced, the plunger is pulled back. If the needle enters the myocardium, the electrocardiogram will show an elevation of the ST segment. Thus an ST segment elevation indicates that the needle has gone too far and is no longer in the pericardial sac. If blood is aspirated with no simultaneous elevation in the ST segment, then the pericardial fluid responsible for the tamponade is most likely being drained.

Blood that has been in the pericardial sac for a period of time will not clot. Therefore, nonclotting blood in the aspirate is another indication of pericardial, rather than ventricular, blood. In the acute

86 situation, even a modest return of only a few cc of blood can produce a rapid elevation in the blood pressure.[15]

Pericardiocentesis may have to be repeated to relieve tamponade recurring prior to transfer to the operating room for thoracotomy. An indwelling catheter inserted through the needle into the peri-cardial sac can provide continuous drain-age if needed.

RUPTURE OF THE AORTA

Rupture of the aorta is usually the result of an abrupt deceleration or compression injury, characteristically an automotive accident.[16] It is often rapidly fatal, and only 10 to 20% of victims survive to reach a hospital.[11, 17] There is no specific therapy that can be applied in the field to reverse the course of the injury, and therefore attempts at diagnosis prior to transport to a hospital are not indicated.

Long-term survival is dependent on prompt diagnosis and treatment in the hospital. Rupture of the aorta is frequently associated with other serious injuries, so a high index of suspicion is needed.[16, 18] On the other hand, in one series, almost one third of patients with aortic rupture had no obvious thoracic injury on initial evalua-tion.[16] The patient may complain of short-ness of breath, chest or back pain and weakness or other abnormalities of the lower extremities, symptoms that are not unique to rupture of the aorta.

The most common site for aortic rupture is the aortic isthmus, distal to the ligamentum arteriosum and the origin of the left subclavian artery.[11] The aorta is relatively fixed at the ligamentum arterio-sum, and the isthmus is thus more subject to stress. The ascending aorta is also relatively frequently involved, with rupture of the descending aorta rarely seen. In about 60% of cases, the aortic adventitia remains intact, which sustains the few survivors of this injury.[18]

The disruption of flow at the site of the rupture accounts for some of the signs associated with aortic rupture. The physi-cal findings of increased blood pressure and pulse amplitude in the upper extremi-ties, coupled with decreased pulse pressure and blood pressure in the lower extremi-ties, although rarely seen, strongly suggest rupture.[16]

The classical radiographic finding in thoracic aortic rupture is widening of the mediastinum. Mediastinal widening, when seen on a postero-anterior chest film, with a patient in a good vertical position, carries a high correlation with rupture.[19, 20] Ficti-tious mediastinal widening can be seen when the patient's position is tilted, or when an antero-posterior projection is used. Mediastinal widening is not pathog-nomonic of aortic rupture, as the widening may be due to bleeding from other mediastinal vessels.[18]

Other radiographic evidence of medias-tinal hematoma, such as deviation of the trachea, compression of the left mainstem bronchus or evidence of major trauma, such as first rib fracture, have been used as predictors of aortic rupture, but do not appear as useful as the detection of a widened mediastinum.[19–21] Ayella, with a series of 36 cases, concluded that the inability to discern the normal superior mediastinal anatomy on an erect chest film should be the basis for diagnosis of mediastinal hematoma.[18] A mediastinal hematoma implies a possible aortic rupture.

Diagnosis of aortic rupture is confirmed with aortography, and a positive aortogram mandates thoracotomy. If there is some delay in the definitive treatment for aortic rupture, the medical management is similar to that of dissecting aneurysm. Hypotensive agents, such as nitroprusside, are used to limit the progression of the rupture until the patient is taken to the operating room.

MYOCARDIAL CONTUSION

Most any blunt force applied to the chest can affect the heart. Forceful chest contact against a steering wheel is the most common cause of myocardial contusion, but the heart can be contused against the sternum with any sharp deceleration.[22, 23] The diagnosis of myocardial contusion is difficult to make, because there are no specific symptoms or findings, and the patient may be completely asymptomatic. The most consistent finding in a patient with myocardial contusion is a tachycardia in the absence of hypovolemia or hypoxia.[23] There may be the imprint of a steering wheel, or other ecchymoses, on the anterior chest. Injuries such as fractured sternum are concomitant with myocardial contusion, but the contusion can occur without any external injury.

Electrocardiographic changes can resemble those of myocardial ischemia and infarction, including ST-T changes, conduction abnormalities and almost any arrhythmia.[18, 23] Unfortunately, the standard 12-lead electrocardiogram may be completely normal, or may become abnormal only after two to four days. Schick has shown that, in experimental myocardial contusion, abnormalities appear in a special high-frequency electrocardiogram, even when the standard electrocardiogram is normal.[22]

The electrocardiogram is still the most reliable way of detecting myocardial contusion, even with its limitations. All patients with known chest trauma should have an electrocardiogram. Any electrocardiographic abnormality, or other evidence of myocardial injury, such as pericardial friction rub, is assumed to be caused by contusion. Since the electrocardiographic abnormalities may not occur for two to four days, if at all, serial electrocardiograms may be needed for that period of time.

The treatment of myocardial contusion is essentially the same as that of myocardial infarction, with hospitalization and electrocardiographic monitoring. Treatment is specific for complications as they occur. The typical course, in the absence of coronary arterial injury, is complete resolution, with electrocardiographic changes resolving in 30 days or less. Most cases of myocardial contusion are probably missed and are only found when late sequelae, such as ventricular aneurysm, are detected.[23, 24]

Rarely, a true myocardial infarct may occur because of blunt injury to coronary vessels.[25]

88 ESOPHAGEAL INJURIES

The esophagus is well protected from most thoracic trauma, as it is deep in the mediastinum, with many surrounding structures. The esophagus may be ruptured by blunt trauma or perforated by missiles or knife wounds. Perforation due to endoscopy is not typically an emergency department case. Traumatic perforation or rupture of the esophagus is as dangerous as it is rare. Untreated, it is nearly 100% fatal. Early diagnosis and repair is essential to avoid a fulminant mediastinitis.[26-29] Esophageal injury may be isolated or masked by other severe trauma.

Approximately 50% of penetrating esophageal injuries occur in the thorax, with most of the remainder occurring in the neck and rarely in the abdominal esophagus.[29] The most common complaints associated with esophageal injury include: pain, coughing, choking, hematemesis, hoarseness, dysphagia, dyspnea and upper abdominal pain. Physical findings, depending on the extent and location of the injury, may include fever (usually occurring within a few hours), contusions, subcutaneous emphysema, mediastinal crunching sounds ("Hamman's sign"), stridor and decreased breath sounds.[26-32] Cyanosis or shock inconsistent with the apparent degree of thoracic trauma, should suggest esophageal injury. The location of the missile or knife wound does not preclude esophageal damage, as esophageal perforation has been reported from wounds lateral to the mid-clavicular line of the chest.[26]

The chest radiograph may show mediastinal widening, pneumomediastinum, pleural effusion, hydropneumothorax, rib fractures, pulmonary contusion, atelectasis, subcutaneous emphysema or foreign bodies.

The diagnosis of esophageal perforation or rupture is accurately made by contrast studies. There is some controversy over the exact contrast agent to use. The injury is more reliably seen using a nonwater-soluble material, such as barium, but the extravasation of such material complicates surgery, as it cannot be left in the mediastinum. Water-soluble material, such as gastrograffin, is slightly less reliable in detecting perforation but is not toxic if extravasated into the mediastinum. One approach is to use gastrograffin initially, and repeat the study with barium if the first study is negative or equivocal.[29]

The initial treatment of esophageal perforation consists of a nasogastric tube for constant suction and the administration of broad spectrum antibiotics. Cephalosporins are reportedly useful.[29] Immediate operative repair is required.

RUPTURE OF THE BRONCHUS

Rupture of a bronchus is an uncommon injury. Its rarity alone makes for an elusive diagnosis.[11,33] Yet it must be suspected with any chest injury, as its initial manifestations may be subtle.

Pneumothorax is common, but a ruptured bronchus can occur without apparent pneumothorax.[11,33,34] A pneumothorax, particularly a tension pneumothorax, that does not respond to a properly inserted thoracostomy tube is essentially diagnostic of ruptured bronchus.[11,33,34]

Hemoptysis is strongly suggestive of

bronchial tear, but it is not a common symptom.[33, 34] A deterioration in the patient's condition, disproportionate to the radiographic or physical findings, may be the only clinical feature of bronchial rupture.

Fracture of at least one of the first three ribs has been noted in almost 90% of bronchial fractures.[5] Therefore, an upper rib fracture compels the consideration of bronchial injury.

Mediastinal or cervical emphysema may be the only radiographic findings. With complete rupture of the mainstem bronchus, a pneumothorax may be seen in which the location of the collapsed lung changes with the patient's position. Since the lung has lost its mechanical support, it assumes a dependent position. Thus, in an upright frontal radiograph, the lung appears on the diaphragmatic surface, rather than perihilar as seen in a simple pneumothorax.[5]

Bronchoscopy is the most effective tool to confirm the diagnosis of acute bronchial rupture. Once the precise nature of the airway injury is defined, the decision on the surgical approach can be made.[11, 33, 34]

RUPTURE OF THE DIAPHRAGM

Diaphragmatic injury usually occurs in the multiply injured patient, and the incidence is markedly increased with pelvic fracture. Although diaphragmatic rupture is associated predominantly with abdominal trauma, it has a reasonable association with thoracic trauma.[11, 35]

Several hypothetical mechanisms have been proposed for rupture of the diaphragm:[11, 35]

1. tearing of the diaphragm as a consequence of respiratory effort by a diaphragm fixed by a crushing force;
2. bursting, due to a sudden severe rise of intra-abdominal pressure relative to intrathoracic pressure;
3. powerful contraction of the diaphragm at the time of injury, causing large avulsion tears; and
4. peripheral tears, caused by perforation and laceration from rib fragments.

Diaphragmatic rupture may be asymptomatic, or the patient may suffer severe pain and respiratory distress. The immediate consequence of symptomatic diaphragmatic rupture is herniation of abdominal contents into the chest, which may compress the lung and in extreme cases compress the mediastinum. This situation can mimic tension pneumothorax, since herniated viscera may rapidly distend and cause tamponade of the lungs and cardiovascular structures. Paradoxical motion of the abdominal organs during inspiration may further complicate the picture. Since at least 60% of normal respiratory effort is dependent on the function of the diaphragm, a large diaphragmatic rent may reduce ventilation by 25% without any herniation.[11] Obstruction of, or hemorrhage into, herniated abdominal viscera may further compromise the patient's status.

Between 80 and 90% of diaphragmatic ruptures occur on the left, possibly because the solid tissue of the liver protects the right side and because of relative weakness of the left posterolateral diaphragm.[5, 11, 35]

The difficulty in diagnosing rupture of the diaphragm is emphasized by the following categorization. Phase one is the initial phase and includes all cases diagnosed within the first month of injury. If the injury is not diagnosed, either because it is asymptomatic or misdiagnosed, the second, or interval, phase is entered. This phase may last from days to years and may be asymptomatic or punctuated by intermittent attacks of pain, possibly caused by incarceration of herniated viscera. In one series, almost half the patients were in phase two, indicating that the diagnosis was not made on initial presentation. Phase three is marked by obstruction and strangulation of the herniated viscera, respiratory distress or both.[35]

About one third of patients may initially be asymptomatic. The most common complaints are abdominal pain, possibly radiating to the shoulder, and dyspnea. Physical findings include a scaphoid abdomen. The presence of bowel sounds in the chest is pathognomonic. Mediastinal shift to the side opposite the rupture is attributed to the loss of negative intrathoracic pressure above the injury and may present as a shift in the trachea or in the area of cardiac percussion dullness. Percussion of the affected chest may be dull or tympanitic, depending on the nature of the herniated viscera.

Plain x-ray studies, preferably an upright chest film, may show any of several signs. Rupture of the left diaphragm appears as:

- an arch-like shadow, mimicking a high left diaphragm;

- extraneous shadows appearing above the typical level of the diaphragm;
- a shift of the heart and mediastinum to the right;
- atelectasis above the aforementioned arch-like shadow;
- air-fluid levels from herniated viscera.

An apparent large left pneumothorax may actually be a distended, herniated stomach, for which a chest tube is inappropriate.

Most ruptures of the right diaphragm are radiographically detected by signs of herniation of the liver. Apparent elevation of the right diaphragm may actually be complete herniation of the liver, in which case an elevation of the inferior edge of the liver may also be noted. A partial herniation of the liver appears as a rounded opacity atop the diaphragm. If other abdominal organs are involved, gas bubbles, air-fluid levels or other opacities may appear.[5, 35]

A nasogastric tube that coils in the left thorax confirms the diagnosis. If the tube cannot be passed into the stomach, contrast agents may show obstruction due to kinking of viscera at the hernial orifice.

The initial management of diaphragmatic rupture is oriented toward the respiratory symptoms. Intubation and mechanical ventilation may be required if the loss of diaphragmatic function is severe.

If a distending herniated stomach is compromising respiration and circulation, decompression with a nasogastric tube is preferred. If the tube cannot be passed, tracheal intubation and mechanical ventilation may provide some relief. If the respiratory compromise is so severe that survival is in doubt, emergency thoracotomy to reduce or decompress the herniated viscus is indicated. Transthoracic catheterization of the distended viscus has been advocated, but this leaves the serious problem of soiling the pleural space with gastrointestinal contents.[35]

Gastrointestinal obstruction and bleeding are treated conventionally with nasogastric suction and fluid replacement.

Diaphragmatic rupture may occur with other injuries, such as ruptured spleen or kidney or multiple rib fractures, and may confuse the diagnosis. Some advocate peritoneal lavage routinely in this situation to evaluate abdominal integrity.[3] Peritoneal lavage fluid in the chest tube drainage is diagnostic of diaphragmatic perforation or rupture.[9]

PENETRATING CHEST WOUNDS

The incidence of penetrating chest wounds is rising.[9, 15] Although most penetrating chest wounds are localized, thoracic gunshot wounds have associated abdominal injuries in 20% of the cases. Knife wounds of the chest carry an 11% incidence of intra-abdominal injury. Any penetrating chest wound at or below the fifth intercostal space may involve the abdomen.

If a patient with a penetrating chest wound arrives in the emergency department with hypotension or strong indication of pneumothorax or hemothorax, a chest tube should be inserted on the affected side. Waiting for a chest x-ray in such cases is unjustified and only permits more bleeding and deterioration.

The incidence of hemothorax or hemopneumothorax is 90% in gunshot wounds of the chest and more than 70% in stab wounds.[2, 10] Thus a large-bore chest tube should be used for penetrating thoracic injury. Since the incidence of hemothorax from thoracic gunshot wounds is so high, and the pulmonary injury and bleeding so great, chest tubes should generally be inserted into the affected chest in all cases, regardless of the patient's apparent condition. The only exception is when strong evidence indicates there was no intrapleural penetration by the missile. For example, when the bullet can be palpated subcutaneously or external evidence of the bullet track precludes penetration, the patient need not be treated so aggressively.

Since a stab wound generally causes less injury and bleeding than a bullet wound, an apparently stable stabbing victim can be evaluated more deliberately and appropriate x-rays obtained. A knife imbedded in the chest wall should not be removed in the field or in the emergency department, as it may be all that is plugging a hole in a blood vessel.

Penetrating wounds of the heart are most often due to knife wounds, but the incidence of gunshot wound has been increasing. A patient with a heart wound will usually be hypotensive, tachycardic and dyspneic. About 80% have a precordial or parasternal wound.[7, 36] Distended neck veins, marking the elevated central venous pressure of pericardial tamponade, are likely to be present, as are muffled heart sounds. However, distended neck veins may not be present, even with tamponade, if the patient is hypovolemic from blood

92

loss and may only appear after vigorous volume restoration.[36]

Initially, treatment consists of fluid replacement. If fluid does not reverse the hypotension, the neck veins distend or the central venous pressure rises above 14 cm of water, pericardiocentesis is indicated. Chest tubes may be required for concomitant pulmonary injury.

If initial treatment does not stem the blood loss or improve the patient's condition, there is likely to be major injury to the heart, great vessels or intercostal or internal mammary arteries. If the rapid infusion of fluids does not support the patient adequately enough to get to the operating room, thoracotomy in the emergency department is indicated. Emergency department thoracotomy is designed for the patient who does not respond to advanced life support therapy. Such a patient's chance of survival, without aggressive intervention, is nil.

The patient must be intubated prior to the procedure. No anesthesia is needed, as the procedure is not undertaken in a conscious patient. The incision should be made in the fourth intercostal space, on the affected side, avoiding the neurovascular structures on the underside of the fourth rib. The procedure cannot be usefully performed without a pair of rib spreaders to widen the intercostal space.

Bleeding from intercostal or internal mammary arteries can be controlled by clamping and ligating. Injuries to larger vessels may be treated by oversewing the hole, if it is small enough, or by direct pressure.

Bleeding from a penetrating wound of the heart can often be initially controlled by blocking the hole with a finger and by applying pressure to the wound without undue compression of the heart. The wound can then be sutured using 2–0 silk on a long thin needle. Horizontal mattress sutures are used, inserted 4 to 6 mm from the wound edge. Teflon pledgets should be used to pad the external loop of thread to prevent tearing of the myocardium. (See Figure 2.) The sutures should be tied just tightly enough to stop the bleeding. If the wound is near a coronary artery, the sutures should be placed deep to the vessel, so that it will not be ligated.

There is some controversy over emergency department thoracotomy. Some believe that thoracotomy should not be performed in community hospital emergency departments and that all serious injuries should be directed to the local county hospital or trauma center, where there is greater expertise.[37] Undoubtedly,

FIGURE 2. USE OF HORIZONTAL MATTRESS SUTURES AND TEFLON PLEDGETS

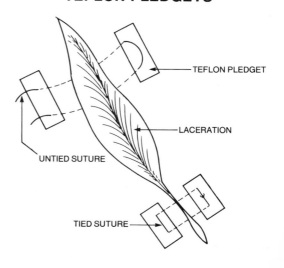

TEFLON PLEDGET

LACERATION

UNTIED SUTURE

TIED SUTURE

the trauma center is better able to handle chest injuries and emergency thoracotomy. However, many parts of the country do not have trauma centers, and there are now skilled, experienced emergency physicians in many community emergency departments. Thus it is not unlikely that a lethally injured patient will present to a community hospital emergency department in which there is a physician with the knowledge required to perform a thoracotomy.

The techniques are relatively straightforward, and the procedure is reserved for the patient who would otherwise die. Clearly some patients can be saved by emergency department thoracotomy, and it is therefore a part of the emergency medicine clinician's armamentarium.[38]

Asymptomatic patients with missile or stab wounds to the chest must be treated expectantly. Even in the absence of apparent intrathoracic injury, pneumothorax or hemothorax may develop in 24 to 48 hours.[9] Hospitalization is indicated unless the wound is clearly nonpenetrating.

Potentially penetrating wounds of the abdomen in asymptomatic patients have been evaluated with local dissection to determine if the wound penetrated peritoneum. Such local dissection is inappropriate in the evaluation of chest wounds, as the procedure may open a sealed tract and precipitate a pneumothorax.[3]

SUMMARY

The incidence of chest trauma is on the rise and continues to be associated with high mortality and morbidity. With the increasingly sophisticated intervention of field emergency medicine clinicians, seriously injured patients are more often reaching the hospital alive. With knowledge of the signs, symptoms and physiological dysfunctions associated with chest injury, and skill in treatment procedures, clinicians will be able to greatly reduce that morbidity and mortality.

REFERENCES

1. Dougall A, et al: Chest trauma—Current morbidity and mortality. *J Trauma* 17:547–553, July 1977.
2. Oparah S, Mandal A: Penetrating gunshot wounds of the chest in civilian practice: Experience with 250 consecutive cases. *Brit J Surg* 65:45–48, January 1978.
3. Thal E: Evaluation of peritoneal lavage and local exploration in lower chest and abdominal stab wounds. *J Trauma* 17:642–648, August 1977.
4. London P: Introduction, in Williams W, Smith R (eds), *Trauma of the Chest*. Bristol, John Wright and Sons, 1977, pp 8–13.
5. Paredes S, Hipona F: The radiologic evaluation of patients with chest trauma. *Med Clin N Amer* 59:37–63, January 1975.
6. Symbas P.: Chest and heart injuries, in Schwartz G, et al (eds): *Principles and Practice of Emergency Medicine*. Philadelphia, WB Saunders Co, 1978, pp 653–673.
7. Siemens R, et al: Indications for thoracotomy following penetrating thoracic injury. *J Trauma* 17:493–500, July 1977.
8. Levinsky L, et al: Thoracic injuries in the Yom Kippur war. Experience in a base hospital. *Isr J Med Sci* 11:275–280, February 1975.
9. Oparah S, Mandal A: Penetrating stab wounds of the chest: Experience with 200 consecutive cases. *J Trauma* 16:868–872, November 1976.
10. O'Riordan W: Autotransfusion in the emergency department of a community hospital. *JACEP* 6:233–237, June 1977.
11. Wilson R, et al: Nonpenetrating thoracic injuries. *Surg Clin N Amer* 57:17–36, February 1977.
12. Trinkle J, et al: Management of flail chest without

94

mechanical ventilation. *Ann Thorac Surg* 19:355–363, April 1975.

13. Trinkle J: Flail chests—Facts and fantasies, in Williams W, Smith R (eds): *Trauma of the Chest.* Bristol, John Wright and Sons, 1977, pp 37–50.

14. Shackford S, et al: The management of flail chest. Comparison of ventilatory and nonventilatory treatment. *Am J Surg* 132:759–762, December 1976.

15. Asfaw I, Arbulu A: Penetrating wounds of the pericardium and heart. *Surg Clin N Amer* 57:37–48, February 1977.

16. Davidson K: Closed injuries to the aorta and great vessels, in Williams W, Smith R (eds): *Trauma of the Chest.* Bristol, John Wright and Sons, 1977, pp 69–79.

17. Freeark R: Blunt torso trauma. *Surg Clin N Amer* 57:1317–1333, December 1977.

18. Ayella R, et al: Ruptured thoracic aorta due to blunt trauma. *J Trauma* 17:199–205, March 1977.

19. Hipona F, Paredes S: The radiologic evaluation of patients with chest trauma—Cardiovascular system. *Med Clin N Amer* 59:65–93, January 1975.

20. Shackford S: The significance of chest wall injury in the diagnosis of traumatic aneurysms of the thoracic aorta. *J Trauma* 18:493–497, July 1978.

21. Marsh D, Sturm J: Traumatic aortic rupture: Roentgenographic indications for angiography. *Ann Thorac Surg* 21:337–340, April 1976.

22. Schick T, et al: Detection of cardiac disturbances following thoracic trauma with high-frequency analysis of the electrocardiogram. *J Trauma* 17:419–424, June 1977.

23. Pearce W, Blair E: Significance of the electrocardiogram in heart contusion due to blunt trauma. *J Trauma* 16:136–140, February 1976.

24. Berkoff H, et al: Asymptomatic left ventricular aneurysm: A sequela of blunt chest trauma. *Circulation* 55:545–548, March 1977.

25. Oren A, et al: Acute coronary occlusion following blunt injury to the chest in the absence of coronary atherosclerosis. *Am Heart J* 92:501–505, October 1976.

26. Popovsky J, et al: Gunshot wounds of the esophagus. *J Thorac Cardiov Surg* 72:609–612, October 1976.

27. Triggiani E, Belsey R: Oesophageal trauma: Incidence, diagnosis, and management. *Thorax* 32(3):241–249, June 1977.

28. Lyons W, et al: Rupture and perforation of the esophagus: The case for conservative management. *Ann Thorac Surg* 25:346–350, April 1978.

29. Defore W Jr, et al: Surgical management of penetrating injuries of the esophagus. *Am J Surg* 134:734–738, December 1977.

30. Symbas P, et al: Penetrating wounds of the esophagus. *Ann Thorac Surg* 13:552–558, June 1972.

31. Sawyers J, et al: Esophageal perforation. *Ann Thorac Surg* 19:233–238, March 1975.

32. Chilimindris C: Rupture of the thoracic esophagus from blunt trauma. *J Trauma* 17:968–971, December 1978.

33. Bates M: Rupture of the bronchus, in Williams W, Smith R (eds): *Trauma of the Chest.* Bristol, John Wright and Sons, 1977, pp 142–150.

34. Guest J, Anderson J: Major airway injury in closed chest trauma. *Chest* 72:63–66, July 1977.

35. Harley H: Traumatic diaphragmatic hernia due to blunt injury, in Williams W, Smith R (eds): *Trauma of the Chest.* Bristol, John Wright and Sons, 1977, pp 80–141.

36. Szentpetery S, Lower R: Changing concepts in the treatment of penetrating cardiac injuries. *J Trauma* 17:457–461, June 1977.

37. Mattox K: Editorial—Emergency department thoracotomy. *JACEP* 7:455, December 1978.

38. MacDonald J, McDowell R: Emergency department thoracotomies in a community hospital. *JACEP* 7:423–428, December 1978.

Abdominal Trauma

Michael C. Tomlanovich, M.D.
Director Residency Program
Division of Emergency Medicine

Richard M. Nowak, M.D.
Senior Staff Physician
Division of Emergency Medicine

Joe G. Talbert, M.D.
Senior Staff Physician
Division of Trauma Surgery

Robert S. Brown, M.D.
Division Head
Division of Trauma Surgery
Henry Ford Hospital
Detroit, Michigan

THE DEATH RATE from trauma has risen from seventh position in 1900 to fourth in 1970, and now accounts for approximately 55 deaths per 100,000 population.[1] It is the number one cause of death in the first three decades of life.[2] Although it is difficult to ascertain the incidence of all types of abdominal trauma, blunt abdominal injuries account for about 1% of all trauma-related hospital admissions.[3] The mortality rate is less than 5% for penetrating injuries of the abdomen[4,5] and between 10 and 30% for blunt injuries.[6-8] The higher mortality statistics for blunt trauma are related to more severe patterns of organ damage, especially of the liver and pancreas, the increased frequency of extra-abdominal injuries and errors in diagnosis.[8,9]

Trauma patients require rapid categorization according to injuries that are immediately life threatening, not immediately life threatening or not readily detectable. This assessment is determined by the clinical status of the patient and may be

96

TABLE 1

Etiological Classification of
Abdominal Trauma

Penetrating Injuries:
  Stab wounds
  Impalement injuries
  Gunshot wounds
  Shotgun wounds
  Shrapnel and flying missiles
Nonpenetrating Injuries:
  Blunt trauma
  Crush injuries
  Seat belt injuries
  Blast injuries
Iatrogenic injuries from emergency
    procedures:
  Cardiopulmonary resuscitation
  Tube thoracostomy
  Peritoneal lavage

aided by understanding the mechanism of injury. (See Table 1.)

PENETRATING ABDOMINAL INJURIES

Penetrating wounds of the abdomen may include all truncal injuries that occur below the fourth intercostal space. However, with penetrating gunshot wounds to any part of the trunk or proximal extremities, the bullet may ricochet off bones and cause possible intra-abdominal penetration. This should be suspected if no exit wound or missile can be located.

In the authors' experience, the number of gunshot wounds exceeds the number of stabbings. However, coincident with the recent passage of tough legislation concerning the criminal use of firearms, the number of stabbings has now increased.

The incidence of organ injury from

penetrating abdominal wounds has been derived from a compilation of nine series, which totalled 3,162 patients with 1,623 positive laparotomies. (See Table 2.) The average number of organ injuries per patient was 1.4. The liver, being the largest intra-abdominal organ, was most often penetrated. The average number of small-bowel perforations per patient was approximately 5.5.[3]

The immediate death from penetrating abdominal trauma is directly related to injury to major vascular structures with resultant intra-abdominal exsanguinating hemorrhage. Otherwise, the mortality directly relates to the number of abdominal organs injured, predisposing medical conditions and the patient's age.

Abdominal Stab Wounds

If at all possible, the emergency clinician should determine the size, shape and length of the stabbing instrument to esti-

TABLE 2

Frequency of Organ Injury in
Penetrating Abdominal Trauma

Organ Injured	% Incidence
Liver	37
Small bowel	26
Stomach	19
Colon	16.5
Major vascular and retroperitoneal	11
Mesentery and omentum	9.5
Spleen	7
Diaphragm	5.5
Kidney	5
Pancreas	3.5
Duodenum	2.5
Biliary system	1
Other	1

mate the potential intra-abdominal damage. In general, the site of a stab wound relates to the organ injured. However, the intra-operative findings may show entirely unsuspected and anatomically unrelated penetration sites. In one series of 371 abdominal stab wounds, 20% were multiple and approximately 10% involved both chest and abdomen.[10] In another series of 550 abdominal stabbings, only three wounds occurred in the back with the remainder located anteriorly and in the flank areas. Most wounds occurred on the left side (compatible with the fact that most assailants would be right handed), and three times as many wounds were located in the upper abdominal quadrants (including the lower costal margin areas) than in the lower quadrants.[11]

Injury to the skin and subcutaneous tissues is usually insignificant, requiring simple wound cleansing with or without primary closure. Penetration of the skin in the abdominal region is not absolute evidence of internal injury.[12] Nearly one third of abdominal stab wounds never penetrate the peritoneal lining. Approximately half of those that enter the peritoneal cavity may not require surgery. The Nance study of 1,180 patients with stab wounds of the abdomen indicated that liver injuries dropped in frequency (probably caused by selected observation of patients with trivial liver injuries not requiring surgical repair), and small bowel lacerations were the most commonly encountered injury.[4]

Impalement Injuries

Impalement injury is an extremely dirty form of stab wound. Impalement injuries secondary to falls from heights tend to occur in the anorectal area, as the anus is at the apex of a funnel whose walls consist of the coccyx, ischial tuberosities and pubis. Consequently, trauma to this area usually results in injury of the anus, rectum and sigmoid colon, with high mortality caused by bacterial contamination.[13] Impaled objects should only be removed in an operating room.

Gunshot Wounds

The seriousness of gunshot wounds is often thought to be caused directly by the bullet. However, the wounding potential of missiles is exceedingly complex and is related to both velocity and bullet mass. This is best understood when one considers that tissue damage is directly proportional to the kinetic energy delivered to the body, i.e., the kinetic energy of the missile entering the body minus that exiting. Kinetic energy is expressed by the formula: $E = (MV^2 \div 2G) \times 7,000$ where E equals energy in foot pounds, M equals mass of the missile in grains, V equals velocity in feet per second, G equals gravitational acceleration in feet per second, and 7,000 being a conversion factor. Thus, kinetic energy is proportional to the mass of the missile and more importantly to the square of its velocity.[3,14]

Most civilian gunshot wounds are of low-muzzle velocity (500 to 1000 feet per second) whereas most military rifles are high-velocity injuries (2000 to 3000 feet per second). The impact velocity will depend on the ballistics of the shell and the distance of the target from the muzzle. This emphasizes the importance of history taking in regard to type of firearm and certainly the distance from which the patient was shot.[15]

Bullet wounding from high-velocity firearms is important because as the missile passes through tissue, a temporary cavity is formed. The size of the cavity is directly proportionate to the energy absorbed by the expanding medium.[14] For this reason, a bone that is not directly struck by a projectile may be fractured from the explosive cavitational effect alone. This, of course, also applies to intra-abdominal organs, either hollow or solid. Additionally, a negative pressure is created, which can draw external debris into the cavity. Hence, high-velocity wounds should be considered contaminated and require debridement.

Tissue characteristics also influence the type of injury, especially at medium- and high-impact velocity. The damage is proportionately greater with increasingly solid tissue, the lungs, skin and fascia reveal little devitalization when struck by missiles whereas solid tissue such as bone, liver and spleen are more significantly damaged.[6] A further point to remember is that missiles may fragment, especially on striking bone, with resultant multiple missiles tracking in different directions causing injury to other intra-abdominal contents. In general, exit wounds are larger than entrance wounds, due to the increased area of the striking surface of a bullet at the point of exit secondary to deformation, yawing or tumbling on passage through the body. In a bullet wound at very close range, the entrance wound may be larger than the exit because the gases in the blast contribute to the surface tissue damage.[16]

In the Nance series, the incidence of abdominal injury from gunshot wounds was strikingly higher (81.6%) than from stab wounds (33%). The mortality rate from gunshot wounds was 12.5% compared to 1.4% for stab wounds. Mortality rate was highly correlated with the number of abdominal organs involved. In descending order the organs injured among their 1,032 patients with gunshot wounds were: small bowel, liver, colon, stomach, kidney, spleen, pancreas, great vessels, duodenum, gallbladder and bladder. Hollow-viscus injury comprised more than half the total, but by itself was seldom a cause of death.[4] Mortality was most frequently related to hemorrhage.

Shotgun Wounds

Shotguns are smooth-bore long-barrelled guns that were designed primarily for killing game birds and small animals. A shotgun wound is caused by many small pellets. Injury is determined by the type and amount of powder charge, the size of pellets, the constriction at the muzzle end of the barrel (choke) and especially the distance from the victim. At a range of ten yards, approximately 95% of these pellets will be within a pattern nine inches in diameter when fired from a full-choke bore (and within an 18-inch circle when fired from a cylinder barrel). At 20 yards these wound diameters are doubled. The unfavorable ballistic characteristics of spheres cause a rapid fall-off of pellet velocity. Thus, the shotgun becomes ineffective at producing severe wounds at long ranges from loss of velocity and dispersion of the pellets.[17]

Accordingly, Sherman and Parrish have described three types of shotgun wounds.

Type one wounds penetrate only subcutaneous tissue or deep fascia and occur at a range greater than seven yards. Type two wounds penetrate beneath the deep fascia and are from blasts at a distance of three to seven yards. Type three injuries are extremely critical and result from shots fired at point blank range, under three yards. Type three wounds may contain the wad and plastic cups used to separate the powder charge from the shot.[18] Tissue damage is proportional to the specific gravity of the tissue hit and inversely proportional to its elastic content. Thus a close-range shotgun blast may cause extensive damage to the liver but relatively less to the adjacent lung.[19]

Type one wounds to the abdomen are treated nonsurgically with antibiotics, tetanus toxoid and appropriate wound care. The management of type two wounds is controversial. With scattered penetrating pellets in the abdomen, Bell has advocated nonoperative management feeling that the small holes in the intestines caused minimal leakage and limited peritonitis and closed spontaneously; furthermore he postulated that mechanical manipulation could cause more leaking and increase contamination.[20] Others have advocated laparotomy in all penetrating shotgun wounds of the abdomen because of possible tangential lacerating wounds to the intestinal mucosa requiring closure. Mortality in type two shotgun wounds to the abdomen is approximately 5%.[18]

The mortality reported by Sherman and Parrish for type three abdominal shotgun wounds was 38.5% (13 cases). Mortality is related to both the massive destructive effects of the pellets on the skin and subcutaneous tissues with resultant closure problems and the multiple and severe organ damage. However, in retrospect some patients with type three shotgun wounds could be better managed with more aggressive fluid and blood therapy.[18] The concept of rapid volume replacement is of paramount importance for the emergency clinician. With adequate fluid therapy, patients may survive to go to the operating room for extensive tissue debridement. Delayed mortality usually results from peritonitis and sepsis.

Mortality from shotgun wounds to the abdomen is estimated to be double that of gunshot wounds.[18, 20] However, statistics relative to the mortality of shotgun wounds are almost meaningless because it is impossible to avoid selection of cases. This, of course, is related to the extreme variation of injury produced by the shotgun.

Shrapnel and Flying Missile Wounds

Sixty-five percent of all injuries in Vietnam were caused by fragmentation and secondary missiles from grenades, bombs and land mines.[21] Shrapnel wounds are usually quite large with extensive tissue destruction and fortunately are relatively rare in the civilian population.[3] Industrial explosions, flying missiles from lawnmowers, storms and automobile accidents are potential causes. Multiple fragmentation injuries resemble shotgun wounds whereas a deep-penetrating missile injury resembles an abdominal stab wound.

The Management of Penetrating Injuries of the Abdomen

Before 1960, virtually all surgeons felt that penetrating abdomen trauma required exploratory laparotomy to rule out visceral

100 injury. However, Shafton challenged this concept by recommending exploratory laparotomy only for patients with physical evidence of visceral injury and observation of those patients without.[12] Clinicians who favor mandatory laparotomy cite the unreliability of physical examination in detecting visceral injury.[10, 22, 23] Bull and Mathewson found that 23% of 78 patients with significant intra-abdominal injury had no accompanying physical signs, and 18% of 100 patients with insignificant intra-abdominal pathology had physical evidence of injury. The 100 patients who underwent negative laparotomy had no serious morbidity and no mortality. Consequently, these investigators feel that all patients with penetrating abdominal injuries should be explored because of unreliability of physical examination and the relatively benign nature of negative laparotomy.[24]

The advisability and safety of selective observation for penetrating abdominal stab wounds was reported by Nance; 392 patients with stab wounds of the abdomen who were selectively managed were compared with 432 similar patients who underwent mandatory exploratory laparotomy. The decision to perform laparotomy in the selective observation group was based on: (1) signs of peritoneal injury, (2) unexplained shock, (3) loss of bowel sounds, (4) organ evisceration and (5) positive diagnostic study. Comparison of the two groups revealed that selective observation had reduced: (1) the percentage of negative laparotomy from 53 to 11%, (2) the overall complication rate from 14 to 8%, (3) the average hospital stay from 7.8 to 5.5 days and (4) the percentage of

patients subjected to exploration from 95 to 45%. Of the 210 patients who were selectively observed, only 4.8% subsequently required laparotomy, and delay caused no mortality or significant morbidity.[4]

Nance also reviewed 1,032 patients with abdominal gunshot wounds and found that 82% had significant visceral injuries. In retrospect, 97% of these patients could have been identified on admission to the emergency department utilizing the above criteria. Thus, 70% of 138 patients who had negative laparotomy for abdominal gunshot wounds could have been identified by a period of observation. There was no significant morbidity or mortality among 52 patients who were observed and did not undergo exploration. Consequently, Nance feels that the percentage of patients who would be spared a laparotomy is smaller for gunshot wounds than for stab wounds (60% versus 18%), but selective observation could be used effectively and safely for both.[4]

Given the current changing debate regarding management of penetrating abdominal wounds, the emergency physician in assessing physical findings and instituting diagnostic studies plays an instrumental role in the decision of the trauma surgeon whether to operate.

NONPENETRATING INJURIES

Blunt Abdominal Trauma

Patients with blunt trauma to the abdomen are challenging diagnostic problems because of the variety of injuries, presenting complaints and physical findings, and the frequency complicating extra-abdominal injuries. The major cause of blunt abdominal trauma is the automobile. Di Vincenti found that automobile accidents and pedestrian accidents together account for 74% of blunt abdominal trauma, blows to the abdomen 14%, falls 9%, and miscellaneous causes the remaining 3%.[8]

Intra-abdominal viscera are injured by crushing, shearing and bursting forces. Crushing forces may compress an organ against the posterior abdominal wall especially the vertebral bodies. Shearing forces may tear both solid and hollow organs especially at the junction of relatively mobile and fixed segments. Force externally applied to the abdomen may cause sudden increased intraluminal pressure of hollow viscera with resulting organ rupture. The flaccid abdomen of the elderly and the intoxicated is much more prone to injury from external forces. Crushing forces are less withstood by solid viscera accounting for their greater frequency of injury.[3]

In the Di Vincenti series, the overall mortality was 23%. Splenic rupture was easily the most common injury with an overall mortality of 28%. However, when splenic rupture was an isolated injury, the mortality was only 4%. When associated with other injury, mortality rose to 50%. The liver was the second most common site of injury and had an overall mortality of 49% (the highest of any intra-abdominal organ). Ruptured hollow viscus, excluding urinary bladder, was observed in 52 of 518 patients with the small bowel most frequently involved. A ruptured urinary bladder was found in 36 patients, kidney lacerations in 28, ruptured diaphragms in 23 and pancreatic injury in seven. Mortal-

ity was lowest with isolated hollow viscus rupture.[8]

Di Vincenti emphasized that extra-abdominal injury was the most significant factor in increasing mortality. Wilson, in a review of 391 cases of blunt abdominal trauma found a 15% mortality rate in isolated abdominal injury, 58% when associated with head injury and 76% when associated with head injury and coma.[9]

Foley, in reviewing the emergency care of auto accident fatalities, found that six of 43 patients died in the hospital of injuries from which they should have survived (ruptured spleen, liver, retroperitoneal hematoma). In retrospect, the cause was progressive hypovolemia, which was either unrecognized or inadequately treated.[25] This reemphasizes the vital importance of emergency fluid resuscitation in patients with blunt abdominal trauma.

Seat Belt Injuries

Studies have shown a 60% decrease in injury[26, 27] and a 35% reduction in major or fatal trauma[28] with use of automotive restraining devices. Injury is avoided by preventing passenger ejection from the automobile and passenger collision with the car interior. In addition, energy-absorbing plastic reduces deformation of the car and results in occupant deceleration, thereby reducing the chance of injury. However, each type of restraint system has associated injury patterns.

Properly worn, lap seat belts rest low over the anterior iliac spines and should not result in intra-abdominal trauma.[29] However, if improperly positioned above

102

the iliac crest, they cause injury to the abdominal wall and/or abdominal organs. With rapid deceleration, the body is hyperflexed about the axis of the seat belt producing sudden band-like compression of the abdominal contents, which may be quite powerful (at 60 miles per hour the kinetic energy dissipated from a 150-pound body is 18,200 foot pounds per second).[30] In the Williams and Kirkpatrick review of 87 cases of lap belt accident victims, 58% suffered intra-abdominal injury of which 95% involved the intestine and mesentery. These injuries ranged from intestinal contusion to frank perforation. Interestingly, in contrast to other types of blunt trauma, solid organ injury was infrequent. The injury occurs by direct compression of the intestine and its mesentery between the seat belt and posterior abdominal wall or entrapment of a short segment of intestine by the seat belt, creating an acute closed loop obstruction with resultant circumferential bowel transection or perforation.[31]

The "seat belt sign" (contusion, abrasion or ecchymosis across the lower abdomen) occurs in less than one third of the cases of associated intra-abdominal injury.[3] In the Williams and Kirkpatrick series, abdominal tenderness on initial examination was noted in over 50% of the cases with intra-abdominal injury but was either overlooked or masked by associated injuries in the remainder. The difficulty of accurate diagnosis is reflected in the increased morbidity and mortality. When surgery was performed within 12 hours, morbidity and mortality were 12.5% whereas if delayed for more than 12 hours, they rose to 50%.[31]

The shoulder/lap belt was evaluated in 63 patients in the same series. With this restraint, most of the decelerating forces are applied to the sturdy thorax commonly resulting in injuries to the ribs, clavicle or sternum. Intra-abdominal injury is relatively rare. Interestingly, 30% of patients with lap belt restraints suffered head or other injuries, whereas with the shoulder/lap belt, only 1.5% of those injured had additional problems.[29]

INTRA-ABDOMINAL COMPLICATIONS OF EMERGENCY PROCEDURES

In patients undergoing cardiopulmonary resuscitation, compressions of the xiphoid process may cause laceration of the liver.[32, 33] With the resultant intraperitoneal bleeding, a postresuscitative state of hypotension may be misinterpreted as secondary to pump failure. Treatment with pressor agents may cause the oligemic state to deteriorate further. The diagnosis is exceedingly difficult to make but should be entertained particularly if the initial resuscitation was performed by inadequately trained personnel. Artificial ventilation will frequently cause gastric distention especially in children. Several cases of gastric rupture resulting from cardiopulmonary resuscitation have been reported.[33] The presence of bloody gastric aspirate in the postresuscitative period suggests this diagnosis.

A recognized complication of tube thoracostomy is inadvertent penetration of abdominal organs. This can occur in low intercostal space tube placement, during "blind" insertion in a patient with unknown diaphragmatic pathology, and with the use of a trocar. An attempt to drain a small hemothorax by low tube positioning using a trocar resulted in splenic penetration requiring laparotomy. (See Figure 1.)

The complications of peritoneal lavage are potentially life threatening but relatively uncommon. They are related to improper orientation or excessive penetration of the obturator into the peritoneal cavity or failure to observe various contraindications such as a full bladder or a gravid uterus. Caution should be exerted in patients with lower abdominal surgical scars or distended loops of bowel.[34-36] Common complications are perforation of vessels, bowel, urinary bladder and retroperitoneal space.[34, 35, 37]

The aggressive resuscitation of the seriously ill or injured requires various invasive procedures. However, these iatrogenic injuries can further complicate the assessment of the initial trauma and also subject the patient to the risk associated with any surgical procedure.

SPECIFIC INJURIES

Liver

Defore, in reviewing 1,590 cases of liver trauma, emphasized that mortality is more closely related to the amount of intra-abdominal injury than the specific hepatic damage. Mortality was 4.4% in isolated liver injury and progressively increased to 72.9% when five or more associated visceral structures were damaged. Blunt liver trauma is ten times more likely to result in death than penetrating trauma.[38]

A rare complication is traumatic hemo-

FIGURE 1. INTRA-ABDOMINAL PLACEMENT OF A CHEST TUBE WITH SPLENIC PENETRATION

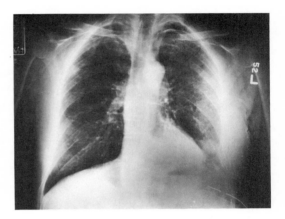

bilia. This presents four to six weeks after liver injury with upper or lower gastrointestinal bleeding, colicky abdominal pain and often obstructive jaundice. This is an important clinical condition to recognize as mortality approaches 100% without appropriate intervention.[39, 40]

Another rare injury secondary to blunt abdominal trauma is disruption of the extrahepatic ductal system. The diagnosis is often difficult and delayed as these patients have a transient chemical peritonitis and may be released from the emergency department. This is followed by a quiescent interval of either days or weeks. Subsequently, the patient presents with jaundice, abdominal tenderness and distention.[41]

Sigmoid Colon and Rectum

Sigmoid colon and rectal injury should be suspected when a penetrating wound occurs in their vicinity even without signs of peritoneal irritation. Leakage from a small perforation may be slow, especially if there is little material in the bowel at the time of injury. Pain is delayed several hours in some cases. Radiographic studies may show intra- or extra-peritoneal gas accumulations.[42] Some recommend diagnostic sigmoidoscopy or contrast studies using diluted Gastrografin.[6] However, Weckesser feels that the diagnosis rests on the clinical impression and a laparotomy is indicated if rectal or sigmoid injury cannot be ruled out.[42]

Spleen

In a review of 408 splenectomies performed for trauma, Naylor reported an overall mortality of 11.2%. However, associated injury was the major factor as no deaths occurred from isolated splenic injury. Mortality was 18.6% for blunt trauma, 8.7% for gunshot wounds and zero for stab wounds. Age was a significant factor as mortality was 40% for patients over 60 and 100% for those over 70.[43]

Delayed splenic rupture has been noted to account for up to one third of all splenic injuries. In this situation, the capsule remains intact, and subcapsular blood accumulates without evidence of intraperitoneal hemorrhage. With further trauma or sudden increased intra-abdominal pressure (e.g., coughing, straining at stool) rupture of the stretched capsule can occur. Some feel that true delayed rupture of the spleen is much less frequent than thought, based on a more aggressive diagnostic evaluation of blunt abdominal trauma utilizing peritoneal lavage and visceral angiography. In a series of 314 patients who underwent splenectomy,

Olsen reported less than a 1% incidence of delayed splenic rupture. Most cases of so-called delayed rupture were actually delayed diagnosis in patients with minimal physical findings from small splenic lacerations with minor bleeding, or larger tears with temporarily contained hemorrhage.[44]

Rib fractures are frequently associated with blunt splenic injury. In children, the flexible rib cage is not often broken but can bend and acts frequently as the causative factor in damaging the spleen.[45]

Pancreas and Duodenum

Pancreatic injuries have been reported in 1 to 2% of all abdominal trauma.[46] The overall mortality rate is 16%: 6% for stab wounds, 15% for gunshot wounds, 61% for shotgun wounds and 16% for blunt trauma. However, Jones and Shires have indicated that mortality rates are primarily due to associated injuries.[47]

The early diagnosis of blunt retroperitoneal duodenal and pancreatic injury continues to be difficult. The classic signs and symptoms of peritoneal irritation are dampened by the retroperitoneal location of these structures. The most common physical finding is minimal epigastric abdominal pain and tenderness, which is present immediately after injury, usually decreases over the next one to two hours, then worsens within six hours. Delayed diagnosis after 24 hours is associated with a marked increase in morbidity and mortality.[48]

Pancreatic trauma is not always associated with hyperamylasemia or an elevated serum amylase. In White's review of 63 patients with pancreatic injury, amylase elevation was present in only 9%

with penetrating trauma and 48% with blunt trauma.[49] To further complicate matters, patients presenting with oligemic shock from other intra-abdominal organ injury may have an elevated serum amylase due to pancreatic ischemia secondary to hypoperfusion alone.[50] However, a rise in serum amylase associated with persistent epigastric tenderness is a significant finding that warrants laparotomy.[48]

Stomach and Small Bowel

Gastric perforations are relatively common in penetrating wounds of the upper abdomen and lower thorax. However, blunt trauma is seldom the cause of significant stomach injury presumably because of its protected location and mobility.[3] Often blood can be aspirated with a nasogastric tube when the stomach has been injured. Injuries to the proximal jejunum and distal ileum (points of relative fixation) are the most common. In a similar manner, adhesions may predispose to localize intestinal tears.[39] The pH of the distal small bowel is often near neutral causing less peritoneal irritation and delayed clinical presentation as compared to the upper jejunum. Paradoxically, the delay in diagnosis is more hazardous because of greater bacterial contamination from the distal ileum.[3]

Abdominal Aorta

It has been estimated that 15% of all patients suffering injury to the abdominal aorta survive long enough to receive medical attention.[51] Beall has reported 14 cases of traumatic aortic disruption with four survivors.[52] With aortic injury, the intact retroperitoneal space can accommodate up to four liters of blood.[3] Patients present with hypotension unresponsive to massive fluid challenge and may require thoracotomy in the emergency department for proximal control of the bleeding site.

Inferior Vena Cava

Inferior vena caval disruption in abdominal trauma occurs approximately once in every 50 cases of gunshot wounds and once in every 300 stabbings. It is very unusual for this injury to be isolated. Importantly, approximately 50% of these patients may clinically present without shock. If present, shock is associated with a marked increase in mortality. Hypovolemic shock is prevented by formation of a retroperitoneal hematoma with spontaneous tamponade. Surgical manipulation of this hematoma can give rise to exsanguinating hemorrhage.[53, 54]

EMERGENCY RESUSCITATION-STABILIZATION

In a severely traumatized patient, survival often hinges on the rapidity of treatment. Therefore, the initial components of any successful resuscitation must be simultaneous diagnosis and treatment of conditions that can produce rapid death. Evaluation of airway patency and ventilatory status must be accompanied by airway management. Determination of blood pressure, pulse rate and presence of external bleeding must be followed by institution of pump support, bleeding control and volume replacement. After stabilization of vital functions, a general assessment should be carried out to estab-

106 lish a comprehensive working diagnosis. Maintenance of a stable state and recognition of new pathology require close monitoring and frequent re-evaluation. The working diagnosis may be confirmed by definitive diagnostic studies. However, time-consuming diagnostic tests can be fatal in an unstable patient whose only salvation lies in immediate surgical intervention.

Respiratory management includes a variety of maneuvers. Supplemental oxygen is necessary for maximal saturation of available hemoglobin. The need for endotracheal intubation or a surgical airway is determined by actual or potential impediments to patency or ventilation.

Hypotension in a patient with abdominal trauma is almost always due to blood loss. A variable number of large-bore intravenous catheters should be placed depending upon the severity of injury. When faced with inadequate peripheral veins, central venous cannulation or deep venous cutdowns are alternatives. In severe hypotensive states, central venous pressure monitoring is an extremely helpful parameter in assessing response to fluid therapy. Under 15 cm of water pressure, the absolute central venous recording is less important than the change in response to volume replacement. With exsanguinating hemorrhage, proximal saphenous vein cutdown with insertion of I.V. extension tubing, allows large-volume infusion at a very rapid rate (500 cc whole blood per five minutes per site). Contrary to Knopp, it is the authors' experience that performance of this cutdown technique is the fastest method of maximal fluid administration.[55] Some question lower extremity approaches in abdominal trauma because of possible inferior vena-caval injuries.[56] As noted previously, this is an uncommon lesion. Even if present, the most aggressive fluid therapy both above and below the site of injury maximizes the resuscitative outcome.

Failure of response to 2000 to 3000 cc of crystalloids suggests massive or ongoing blood loss and indicates the need to additionally institute whole blood transfusion. Massive transfusions require warming and interval administration of bicarbonate calcium, labile clotting factors and platelets. Since laparotomy is not a recommended emergency department procedure, autotransfusion of free peritoneal blood is not currently feasible.

Insertion of a nasogastric tube allows evacuation of gastric contents preventing aspiration, decompresses the gastric dilatation often seen with trauma and permits detection of blood from stomach injury. A Foley catheter is valuable in assessing urinary output as a parameter of adequacy of resuscitation; blood indicates urinary tract injury. However, a spontaneously voided urine is diagnostically preferable.

Antibiotic Use in Abdominal Trauma

Under normal conditions, the large intestine contains a predominantly anaerobic flora consisting of bacteroides, bifidobacteria, peptostreptococci and clostridia having a total concentration of 10^{11} per gram. The small intestine has a relatively sparse indigenous flora with much less anaerobic content.[57] Gastrointestinal perforation from both blunt and penetrating abdominal trauma results in bacterial contamination of the peritoneal cavity. Fullen showed that penetrating wounds treated with antibiotics preoperatively had an infectious complication rate of 7% whereas those treated intra-operatively had a 33% infective rate.[58,59] Most agree that the incidence of infective complications in abdominal trauma can be decreased by the choice and timing of antibiotic administration. Therapy should be initiated as soon as ruptured viscus is suspected. The effective period of preventative antibiotic action in experimental wounds is short, ending within three hours.[60] Antibiotics are markedly less effective in contaminated wounds if administration is delayed more than 12 hours.[61]

In adult patients with suspected intestinal perforation, 2 gm of intravenous cephalothin and 450 mg of intravenous clindamycin are administered. Further maintenance therapy is dependent upon operative findings. As with all penetrating trauma, appropriate tetanus toxoid and hyperimmune gammaglobulin are given.

Military Anti-Shock Trouser (MAST)

Gardner and Ludewig have documented the efficacy of external counterpressure in prolonging survival time of dogs with surgically produced aortic lacerations.[62,63] Clinically, Gardner has shown the beneficial effects of the MAST suit in treating massive abdominal hemorrhage secondary to gynecologic catastrophies, ruptured abdominal aortic aneurysms and other large vessel injuries.[62,64] The usefulness of the device in treating penetrating abdominal trauma from shrapnel and gunshot wounds was demonstrated by Cutler in a study carried out in Vietnam.[65] The value of the MAST suit in penetrating and blunt abdominal trauma with exsanguinating hemorrhage has been well documented.[66]

The MAST device stabilizes the cardiovascular system by applying external circumferential pressure resulting in the autotransfusion of an estimated 1000 ml infradiaphragmatic blood within one to two minutes.[66] The MAST trousers will also prevent or slow blood loss by decreasing transmural pressure of a lacerated vessel. Circumferential compression will decrease the size of a longitudinal vessel laceration, thus further slowing the rate of leakage.[67]

The MAST device is not a substitute for adequate blood volume replacement in treating hemorrhagic shock. It does, however, provide temporary cardiovascular support while other means of resuscitation are being instituted, especially during transport to a medical facility.

Thoracotomy with Thoracic Aortic Occlusion

Since major intra-abdominal vascular laceration has a high mortality rate, some have felt that patients "in extremis" with hypotension refractory to massive fluid challenge and increasing tense abdominal distention require immediate laparotomy. However, laparotomy may result in further circulatory collapse when the release of the abdominal wall tamponade accelerates blood loss. Ledgerwood noted that such patients should be immediately transported to the operating room with continuing aggressive volume replacement. Patients with persistent severe hypo-

108 tension should undergo a left-lateral thoracotomy with clamp occlusion of the descending aorta prior to laparotomy. This approach allows blood pressure restoration to the heart and brain and proximal arterial control of the intra-abdominal bleeding site. In the Ledgerwood study, the duration of aortic occlusion in 11 surviving patients ranged from seven to 60 minutes without the development or progression of neurological deficit.[68]

This protocol for managing exsanguinating intra-abdominal hemorrhage takes advantage of the operating room with proper lighting, sterile technique and skilled personnel. However, patients presenting to the emergency department with abdominal trauma who suffer cardiopulmonary arrest require immediate left-lateral thoracotomy and occlusion of the descending thoracic aorta just above the diaphragm. Institution of internal cardiac massage, volume replacement and correction of acidosis is followed by internal defibrillation and restoration of normal sinus rhythm. Subsequently, the patient is taken to the operating room for definitive laparotomy. Recently, a patient with a gunshot wound to the iliac artery with no obtainable vital signs was treated in this manner, attained a blood pressure of 120/80 and was taken to the operating room.

Furthermore, an arrested patient with penetrating abdominal trauma may have sustained a related concomitant intrathoracic injury. Immediate thoracotomy in this situation allows visualization of the thoracic cavity for tamponade or exsanguinating hemorrhage and appropriate life-saving surgical intervention.

PHYSICAL EXAMINATION

Although only a component of the total patient evaluation, certain physical findings have a positive correlation with intra-abdominal pathologies.

There are several useful points to remember when examining a patient with abdominal trauma:

1. The signs and symptoms in abdominal trauma are a result of blood loss, contusion or laceration of solid organs, and irritating leakage from hollow organs.[3] Solid visceral injuries tend to bleed heavily and lead to early signs of hypovolemia and late signs of peritonitis whereas hollow visceral injuries generally produce the opposite result.[6]

2. The peritoneal cavity extends well above the lower rib margins. Patients with blunt trauma to the lower rib cage or penetrating trauma as high as the fourth or fifth intercostal spaces should be suspect for intra-abdominal injury.

3. Abdominal injuries can be masked in patients with mental obtundation from head injury, intoxication or metabolic derangement. In one series, the mortality rate was four times greater in patients with concomitant head injury and was felt to be due in part to missed diagnosis. In these patients, useful indicators of intra-abdominal injury were absent bowel sounds, abdominal rigidity and unexplained shock.[9] Head injuries do not produce hypotension except in terminal stages, and shock in association

with abdominal trauma is due to abdominal injury until proven otherwise.[3]

4. The incidence of visceral injury from gunshot wounds is much higher than with stab wounds.

5. In most penetrating trauma, patients with intra-peritoneal injury can be distinguished from those with no injury on first evaluation. However, blunt abdominal trauma can cause more subtle organ injuries, and patients may be initially asymptomatic.[4] This was exemplified in a report on blunt duodenal injury in which over 50% of the patients had a delay in diagnosis of over 12 hours.[69]

6. In view of the potential for delayed appearance of signs in abdominal trauma, a high index of suspicion is paramount. It is important to establish baseline physical findings and closely monitor for evolving change.

In alert patients pain is the key symptom. In contrast to the visceral peritoneum, the parietal peritoneum (especially the anterior portion) is richly supplied with sensory nerves. Peritoneal irritation generally gives rise to sharp localizing pain. However, stimulation of the central diaphragmatic peritoneum can lead to pain referred to the ipsilateral shoulder.[70] Patients may complain of left- or right-shoulder pain in splenic (Kehrer's sign) or hepatic injury. Trendelenburg positioning allows irritants to accumulate under the diaphragms and accentuates these symptoms. Referred testicular pain can be seen in retroperitoneal injuries.[3]

The abdomen should be inspected for penetration, evisceration, distention and/or discoloration. Acute abdominal distention usually reflects gastric dilatation or significant peritoneal collection of blood or free air.[71] Ecchymotic discoloration of the flanks (Grey-Turner sign) or umbilicus (Cullen's sign) is occasionally associated with hemorrhage from various retroperitoneal injuries. This tends to be a delayed finding[72] and does not necessarily differentiate between intra- and retroperitoneal bleeding.[73] All patients should be inspected for gross blood in the stomach, rectum and urine. Hematuria is found in most genitourinary injuries.[74] Rectal and gastric blood is not commonly found especially in blunt trauma[7] but is valuable diagnostic information.

Irritation of the peritoneum can cause intestinal paralysis via the peritoneo-intestinal reflex.[75] The auscultatory finding of absent or markedly decreased bowel sounds was found in approximately 90% of instances of visceral injury in one series[76] and totally absent in every patient in another series.[77] However, the presence of bowel sounds does not exclude intra-abdominal injury. Additionally, spinal cord injury and thoracolumbar vertebral fractures can produce adynamic ileus but the possibility of coexistent abdominal pathology should be considered.[9] Bowel sounds in the chest suggest diaphragmatic rupture with bowel herniation.

Abnormal abdominal percussion can be seen with various intra-abdominal injuries. The loss of liver dullness results from bowel perforation with pneumoperitoneum. Loss of gastric tympany in Traube's space can be found in splenic injury (Ballance's sign).[6] Flank dullness that does not change with position suggests retro-peritoneal hematoma.[72]

Abdominal tenderness and guarding to palpation is the most frequent and reliable sign of intra-abdominal injury[7, 8, 71] Abdominal wall contusions produce focal tenderness, but the pain associated with these lesions is generally worsened by exertion of the abdominal wall muscula-ture (as in leg raising against resistance).[6]

The most common etiology of subcuta-neous emphysema is of thoracic origin and thus is the most likely cause when found in the abdominal wall. It can, however, be found in ruptures of the rectum, distal colon, duodenum and any intestine along its mesenteric border.[78]

Abdominal wall rigidity or involuntary guarding is a helpful physical finding and is mediated by a spinal cord reflex initiated from parietal peritoneal irritation.[75] It can also be seen in head injury (and in this instance would be associated with general-ized muscle rigidity), spinal cord irritation, abdominal wall injury and thoracic wall injury.[70] Despite this variability, it is safest to assume that abdominal rigidity is of intra-abdominal origin until it is proven otherwise.

Although uncommon and late occur-ring, abdominal masses are noted in blunt trauma, apparently as a result of subcapsu-lar hepatic or splenic hemorrhage or bleed-ing limited by adhesions, mesentery or omentum.[3, 71] Tender palpable masses are also associated with retroperitoneal hema-tomas.[73] Rupture of the rectus abdominis muscle produces a tender abdominal mass which occurs 80% of the time below the umbilicus. On raising the head against resistance, a subcutaneous mass should

change position, an intraperitoneal mass should disappear and a rectus hematoma remain unchanged (Bouchacourt's sign).[79]

Whenever possible, rectal, genital and pelvic examination should be included in all cases of significant abdominal trauma. A boggy mass anterior to the rectum is associated in some cases of retroperitoneal hematoma[73] and an elevated or nonpalpa-ble prostate is noted with urethral transec-tion above the urogenital diaphragm.[74] Bimanual rectal-vaginal examination can detect blood or air in the cul-de-sac. Retroperitoneal injuries, particularly spinal injuries, can produce priapism.[3] Free penile bleeding and/or a perineal mass are asso-ciated with urethral transection below the urogenital diaphragm.[74]

The major physical signs of diagnostic importance in abdominal trauma include: (1) significant abdominal tenderness; (2) loss of bowel sounds; (3) abdominal rigid-ity; and (4) unexplained shock. Their presence should signal the high likelihood of intra-abdominal injury and prompt needed confirmatory diagnostic studies.

DIAGNOSTIC STUDIES

Laboratory Studies

The most useful tests in evaluating abdominal trauma include a hemoglobin, serum amylase and urinalysis. However, therapeutic decisions are seldom based on their results alone. Typically, the leukocyte count will be elevated from the systemic adrenergic response to trauma. The hemo-globin may be normal or low. It is gener-ally recognized that several hours are required for hemodilution to occur after acute hemorrhage resulting in a normal initial hemoglobin.[56] However, with loss of greater than 20% of blood volume, rapid plasma refill can occur (1000 ml per hour for the first two hours).[80] Thus a low initial hemoglobin may reflect major acute blood loss.

As previously noted, the serum amylase does not correlate well with pancreatic injury. In another series, Olsen reviewed 179 patients with blunt abdominal trauma and found 36 with hyperamylasemia. Only three of these had pancreatic injury.[81]

The absence of blood on urinalysis does not exclude renal injury since up to 20% will not demonstrate microscopic hematuria. Disruption of the renal vasculature or distal ureter can prevent blood from passing into the lower urinary tract.[74, 82] Dark red or burgundy-colored urine which is heme reactive but without RBCs suggests hemoglobinuria or myoglobinuria. The serum in myoglobinemia is normal whereas it is pink in hemoglobinemia. Myoglobinuria is seen with crush injuries, and if severe, may cause renal damage.[83]

Roentgenologic Studies

Stabilized patients require radiologic evaluation including an upright posterior-anterior chest and a supine and left lateral decubitus or upright study of the abdomen. Abnormalities suggestive of intra-abdominal injury are numerous and often subtle, and these x-ray studies should be carefully scrutinized. Important radiographic findings include skeletal fractures with highly associated visceral injuries (e.g., bladder rupture with pelvic fracture), the presence or absence of missiles or foreign bodies (see Figure 2), free intraper-

FIGURE 2. NONEXITING MISSILE FROM A GUNSHOT WOUND TO THE MID ABDOMEN WITH MISSILE RESTING IN THE SCROTUM DEMONSTRATING THE UNPREDICTABILITY OF BULLET TRAJECTORY

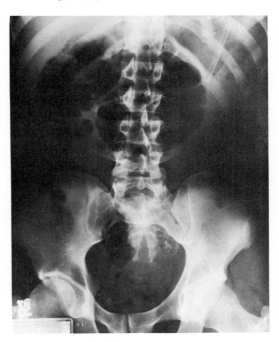

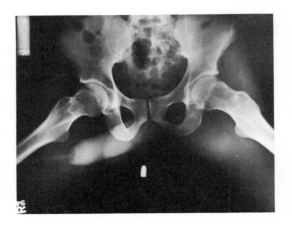

112 itoneal air, retroperitoneal gas accumulations, intraperitoneal fluid, obliteration of psoas shadows (see Figure 3) and enlargement, displacement, or distortion of various hollow or solid viscera.[3]

All stable patients sustaining penetrating or significant blunt trauma to the abdomen with or without hematuria should also have a radiologic evaluation of the urinary tract. This is especially true in children because of the anatomic vulnerability of their urinary tract to injury in blunt trauma.[84] Intravenous pyelography should be performed prior to retrograde cystography as contrast extravasation from

FIGURE 3. ABSENT RIGHT PSOAS SHADOW AND SCOLIOSIS INDICATING RETROPERITONEAL INVOLVEMENT IN A GUNSHOT WOUND TO THE ABDOMEN

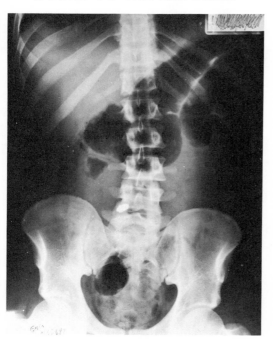

the cystogram can obscure subsequent assessment of the distal ureters. In patients requiring urgent surgical intervention, a bolus-injected two-minute single projection pyelogram is useful in determining contralateral renal function in the event of nephrectomy. With exsanguinating hemorrhage, these studies should be done intra-operatively after hemostasis is achieved.

Cystourethrography is useful in the diagnosis of bladder and urethral tears but there is controversy regarding the value of pyelography in the definitive diagnosis of renal injury.[74] In the absence of shock, unilateral delayed or non-visualization of a kidney is highly suggestive. In this instance, selective angiography can better aid in determining the extent and exact location of a renal injury.

Abdominal arteriography and radionuclide imaging are useful adjunct modalities in stable patients suspected of intra-abdominal injury when the more conventional diagnostic studies are equivocal. These studies have their greatest value in delineating injuries to spleen, kidney, liver and aorta.[85]

Local Wound Exploration

Local exploration of penetrating wounds is advocated by some to lower the rate of negative laparotomy. Peritoneal penetration is not an absolute indication of surgically significant injury. On the other hand, the blast effect associated with high-velocity missiles may cause intra-abdominal damage without peritoneal penetration. The authors prefer not to explore wounds in the emergency department and rely instead upon peritoneal lavage and close clinical observation.

Peritoneal Lavage

During 1978, the authors prospectively studied the efficacy of lavage in 243 patients (121 cases of blunt and 122 cases of penetrating trauma to the lower chest and abdomen). Of 243 lavage procedures, there were three iatrogenic injuries early in the series including two small bowel perforations and a lacerated iliac vein. The lavage was considered positive with: an RBC count of $\geq 100,000/mm,^3$ a WBC count of $\geq 500/mm,^3$ an elevated amylase or the presence of bile or bacteria.

Of the 121 lavages for blunt trauma there were four false positives and three false negatives. Two of the false positives were due to the previously mentioned iatrogenic injuries, and the other two were secondary to retroperitoneal hematomas accompanying pelvic fractures. The three false negatives all occurred with intraperitoneal urinary bladder rupture.

Peritoneal lavage is a standard procedure in the evaluation of blunt abdominal trauma. As seen before, the physical examination and initial clinical impression in blunt injury can be notoriously unreliable.[86] Engrav reported positive peritoneal lavage findings in 20% of patients without peritoneal signs and in only 44% of patients with signs of intra-abdominal injury.[87]

Ahmad and Polk reported a series of 315 patients with blunt trauma studied prospectively by peritoneal lavage with a 97% accuracy rate.[88] More recently Fischer reported a 14–year experience with 2586 patients using lavage to evaluate blunt abdominal trauma and their accuracy was 98.5%.[89] The authors' series in blunt trauma shows 3% false positive and 2% false negative lavages for an overall accuracy rate of 95% which is comparable to other series reported.[90]

A common source of false negative lavage in the authors' experience has been rupture of the urinary bladder. Fortunately these patients present with hematuria, and routine cystography has detected the injury in all cases. Another condition commonly causing false negative lavage is a ruptured hemidiaphragm. In Fischer's large series there were 22 patients with diaphragmatic rupture, and nine of these had a negative lavage for an accuracy rate of 59.1%.[89]

Retroperitoneal hematoma accompanying pelvic fracture has been a source of two of the false positive lavages in the authors' series. It has been the authors' policy to perform arteriography in patients with both positive lavage and pelvic fracture. This procedure can be both diagnostic and therapeutic. First, arteriography allows assessment of the liver, spleen and great vessel integrity. Second, since pelvic fracture has the potential for massive hemorrhage with difficult direct operative control, arteriographic embolization of the bleeding retroperitoneal vessels may be the treatment of choice.[91]

In the authors' series, patients with penetrating trauma to the abdomen and thorax below the fourth intercostal space were screened with peritoneal lavage. Those with obvious injury, however, received immediate rapid resuscitation and operative intervention. Lavage was performed on 56 patients with gunshot wounds. There were 20 true positives, no

114

false positives, 34 true negatives, and two false negatives. It is interesting to note that six laparotomies were performed on clinical grounds in spite of a negative lavage, and all such explorations were negative.

Peritoneal lavage was performed in 66 cases of abdominal stab wounds. There were 15 true positives, one false positive (iatrogenic injury), 48 true negatives, and two false negatives. Again, two laparotomies were performed in the face of a negative lavage, and both were negative.

As a subgroup the authors analyzed 56 lavages performed for isolated penetrating wounds of the thorax. Peritoneal lavage was found to be an excellent tool in detecting unsuspected intra-abdominal injury. There were 14 true positives, one false positive and 41 true negatives.

Peritoneal lavage in the management of penetrating wounds of the abdomen is controversial since historically mandatory exploration has been advocated. However the rate of negative findings in mandatory laparotomy has been disturbingly high. Nance employed peritoneal lavage along with close clinical observation in reducing negative exploration from 53% to 11% in abdominal stab wounds.[4] Thal reported a 4.1% negative laparotomy rate in a series of 123 patients with stab wounds of the lower chest and abdomen investigated by lavage and local wound exploration.[92]

Currently, it is the authors' policy to observe stab wounds of the lower chest and abdomen if there is no clinical evidence of intraperitoneal injury and the peritoneal lavage is negative. The authors followed 66 patients in this fashion with 1.6% false positives, 3.2% false negatives and no mortality in the observed group. All gunshot wounds with apparent intra-abdominal injury are explored promptly. The authors have attempted to evaluate peritoneal lavage findings and correlate them with the patients' clinical course. Lavage has been employed in 56 patients with gunshot wounds to the abdomen and lower thorax with an accuracy rate of 96%. All explorations performed on clinical grounds with negative lavage findings have been negative to date.

SUMMARY

Abdominal injuries span a very broad spectrum of clinical presentations ranging from virtually asymptomatic to frank moribund states. Vascular and solid visceral injuries generally produce acute hemodynamic changes requiring immediate recognition, rapid resuscitation with particular emphasis on volume replacement, and timely surgical hemostasis. However, significant hollow visceral injuries, especially those caused by blunt mechanisms, may be extremely subtle; yet delayed discovery leads to markedly increased morbidity and mortality rates. In this instance, a high index of suspicion is of paramount importance and should prompt a thorough history and physical examination and aggressive judicious diagnostic evaluation. Emergency intervention is a pivotal link in the ultimate outcome of abdominal trauma.

REFERENCES

1. Glacier W: The task of medicine. *Scien Amer* 228:13, 1973.
2. Litwin M, Drapanas T: Trauma: management of the acutely injured patient, in Sabiston D (ed): *Davis-Christopher Textbook of Surgery* ed. 11. Philadelphia, WB Saunders Co, 1977, p 351.
3. Anderson D, Ballinger W: Abdominal injuries, in Ballinger W, Rutherford R, Zuidema G (eds): *The Management of Trauma* ed. 2. Philadelphia, WB Saunders Co, 1973, p 396.
4. Nance F, Wennar M, Johnson L, et al: Surgical judgment in the management of penetrating wounds of the abdomen. *Ann Surg* 179:639, 1974.
5. Pridgen J, Herff A, Watkins H, et al: Penetrating wounds of the abdomen. *Ann Surg* 165:901, 1967.
6. Mackenzie J: Emergency management of trauma to the abdomen, in Schwartz G, Safar P, Stone J, et al (eds): *Principles and Practice of Emergency Medicine.* Philadelphia, WB Saunders Co, 1978, p 673.
7. Davis J, Cohn I, Nance F: Diagnosis and management of blunt abdominal trauma. *Ann Surg* 183:672, 1976.
8. Di Vincenti F, Rives J, Laborde E, et al: Blunt abdominal trauma. *J Trauma* 8:1004, 1968.
9. Wilson C, Vidrine A, Rives J: Unrecognized abdominal trauma in patients with head injuries. *Ann Surg* 161:608, 1965.
10. Maynard A, Oropeza G: Mandatory operation for penetrating wounds of the abdomen. *Am J Surg* 115:307, 1968.
11. Moss L, Schmidt F, Creech O: Analysis of 550 stab wounds of the abdomen. *Am J Surg* 28:483, 1962.
12. Shafton G: Indications for operation in abdominal trauma. *Am J Surg* 99:657, 1960.
13. Wanebo H, Hunt T, Mathewson C: Rectal injuries. *J Trauma* 9:719, 1969.
14. DeMuth W: Bullet velocity and design as determinants of wounding capability: an experimental study. *J Trauma* 6:222, 1966.
15. DeMuth W: Bullet velocity as applied to military rifle wounding capacity. *J Trauma* 9:27, 1969.
16. Fatteh A: *Medicolegal Investigation of Gunshot Wounds.* Philadelphia, JB Lippincott Co, 1976, p 118.
17. DeMuth W: The mechanism of shotgun wounds. *J Trauma* 11:219, 1971.
18. Sherman R, Parrish R: Management of shotgun injuries: a review of 152 cases. *J Trauma* 3:76, 1963.
19. Ledgerwood A: The management of shotgun wounds. *Surg Clin N Amer* 57:111, 1977.
20. Bell M: The management of shotgun wounds. *J Trauma* 11:522, 1971.
21. Howard J, Brown R: Military surgery, in Rhoads J, Allen J, Harkins H, et al (eds): *Surgery: Principles and Practice* ed. 4. Philadelphia, JB Lippincott Co, 1970, p 563.
22. Forde K, Ganepola G: Is mandatory exploration for penetrating abdominal trauma extinct? The morbidity and mortality of negative exploration in a large municipal hospital. *J Trauma* 14:764, 1974.
23. Kazarian K, DiSpaltro F, McKinnon W, et al: Stab wounds of the abdomen: an analysis of 500 patients. *Arch Surg* 102:465, 1971.
24. Bull J, Mathewson C: Exploratory laparotomy in patients with penetrating wounds of the abdomen. *Am J Surg* 116:223, 1968.
25. Foley R, Harris L, Pilcher D: Abdominal injuries in automobile accidents: review of care of fatally injured patients. *J Trauma* 17:611, 1977.
26. Braunstein P: Medical aspects of automotive crash injury research. *JAMA* 163:249, 1957.
27. Lingren S, Warg E: Seat belts in accident prevention. *Practitioner* 188:467, 1962.
28. Tourin B, Garrett J: *Safety Belt Effectiveness in Rural California Automobile Accidents. Automotive Crash Injury Research.* Ithaca, NY, Cornell University, 1960.
29. Sube J, Zipperman H, McIver W: Seat belt trauma to the abdomen. *Am J Surg* 113:316, 1967.
30. Ritchie W, Ersek R, Bunch W, et al: Combined visceral and vertebral injuries from lap type seat belts. *Surg Gynecol Obstet* 131:431, 1970.
31. Williams J, Kirkpatrick J: The nature of seat belt injuries. *J Trauma* 11:207, 1971.
32. Tintinalli J: Cardiopulmonary resuscitation and hypovolemic shock. *J Amer Coll Emerg Physicians* 6:218, 1977.
33. American Heart Association: Standards for cardiopulmonary resuscitation and emergency cardiac care. *JAMA* 227 (suppl), 1974.
34. Sachatello C, Bivins B: Technique for peritoneal dialysis and diagnostic peritoneal lavage. *Am J Surg* 131:637, 1976.
35. Jergens M: Peritoneal lavage. *Am J Surg* 133:365, 1977.
36. Haycock C, Machiedo G: The use of peritoneal lavage as a diagnostic tool in emergencies. *J Amer Coll Emerg Physicians* 3:397, 1974.
37. Breen P, Rudolf L: Potential sources of error in the use of peritoneal lavage as a diagnostic tool. *J Amer Coll Emerg Physicians* 3:401, 1974.

38. Defore W, Mattox K, Jordan G, et al: Management of 1,590 consecutive cases of liver trauma. *Arch Surg* 111:493, 1976.

39. Walt A, Wilson R: Specific abdominal injuries, in Walt A, Wilson R (eds.): *Management of Trauma: Pitfalls and Practice*. Philadelphia, Lea and Febiger, 1975, p 348.

40. Reinhardt G, Hubay C: Surgical management of traumatic hemobilia. *Am J Surg* 121:328, 1971.

41. Zollinger R, Keller R, Hubay C: Traumatic rupture of the right and left hepatic ducts. *J Trauma* 12:563, 1972.

42. Weckesser E, Putnam T: Perforating injuries of the rectum and sigmoid colon. *J Trauma* 2:474, 1962.

43. Naylor R, Coln D, Shires T: Morbidity and mortality from injuries to the spleen. *J Trauma* 14:773, 1974.

44. Olsen W, Polley T: A second look at delayed splenic rupture. *Arch Surg* 112:422, 1977.

45. Ein S: Abdominal injuries, in Salter R (ed): *Care for the Injured Child*. Baltimore, Williams and Wilkins Co, 1975, p 150.

46. Northrup W, Simmons R: Pancreatic trauma: a review. *Surg* 71:27, 1972.

47. Jones R, Shires T: Pancreatic trauma. *Arch Surg* 102:424, 1971.

48. Lucas D: Diagnosis and treatment of pancreatic and duodenal injury. *Surg Clin N Amer* 57:49, 1977.

49. White P, Benfield J: Amylase in the management of pancreatic trauma. *Arch Surg* 105:158, 1972.

50. Warshaw A, O'Hara P: Susceptibility of the pancreas to ischemic injury in shock. *Ann Surg* 188:197, 1978.

51. Yeo M, Domanskis E, Bartlett R, et al: Penetrating injuries of the abdominal aorta. *Arch Surg* 108:839, 1974.

52. Beall A: Penetrating wounds of the aorta. *Am J Surg* 99:770, 1960.

53. Starzl T, Kaupp H, Beheler E, et al: Penetrating injuries of the inferior vena cava. *Surg Clin N Amer* 43:87, 1963.

54. Bricker D, Morton J, Okies J, et al: Surgical management of injuries to the vena cava: changing patterns of injury and newer techniques of repair. *J Trauma* 11:725, 1971.

55. Knopp R: Venous cutdowns in the emergency department. *J Amer Coll Emerg Physicians* 7:439, 1978.

56. Walt A, Wilson R: General considerations in abdominal trauma, in Walt A, Wilson R (eds): *Management of Trauma: Pitfalls and Practice*. Philadelphia, Lea and Febiger, 1975.

57. Thadepalli H, Gorbach S, Broida P, et al: Abdominal trauma, anaerobes, and antibiotics. *Surg Gynecol Obstet* 137:270, 1973.

58. Fullen W, Hunt J, Altemeier W: The time factor in antibiotic prophylaxis of penetrating wounds of the abdomen. *Surg Forum* 22:58, 1971.

59. Fullen W, Hunt J, Altemeier W: Prophylactic antibiotics in penetrating wounds of the abdomen. *J Trauma* 12:282, 1972.

60. Burke J: The effective period of preventive antibiotic action in experimental incisions and dermal lesions. *Surg* 50:161, 1961.

61. Alexander J, Altemeier W: Penicillin prophylaxis of experimental staphylococcal wound infections. *Surg Gynecol Obstet* 120:243, 1965.

62. Gardner W, Storer J: The use of the G-suit in control of intra-abdominal bleeding. *Surg Gynecol Obstet* 123:792, 1966.

63. Ludewig R, Wangensteen S: Aortic bleeding and the effect of external counterpressure. *Surg Gynecol Obstet* 128:252, 1969.

64. Gardner W, Taylor H, Dohn D: Acute blood loss requiring 58 transfusions: the use of the antigravity suit as an aid to post-partum intra-abdominal hemorrhage. *JAMA* 167:985, 1958.

65. Cutler B, Daggett W: Application of the G-suit to the control of hemorrhage in massive trauma. *Ann Surg* 173:511, 1971.

66. Kaplan B, Civetta J, Nagel E, et al: The military anti-shock trouser in civilian pre-hospital emergency care. *J Trauma* 13:843, 1973.

67. Soler J, Muller H, Kennedy T: Clinical use of the G-suit. *J Amer Coll Emerg Physicians* 5:609, 1976.

68. Ledgerwood A, Kozmers M, Lucas C: The role of thoracic aortic occlusion for massive hemoperitoneum. *J Trauma* 16:610, 1976.

69. Lucas C, Ledgerwood A: Factors influencing the outcome after blunt duodenal injury. *J Trauma* 15:839, 1975.

70. Macbeth A: The abdominal wall, umbilicus, peritoneum, mesenteries, and retroperitoneum, in Sabiston D (ed): *Davis-Christopher Textbook of Surgery*. Philadelphia, WB Saunders Co, 1977.

71. Perry J: Blunt and penetrating abdominal injuries. *Curr Prob Surg* May, 1970.

72. McClelland R, Jones R, Shires G, et al: Trauma to the abdomen, in Shires T (ed): *Care of the Trauma Patient*. New York, McGraw-Hill, 1966, p 354.

73. Baylis S, Lansing E, Glas W: Traumatic retroperitoneal hematoma. *Am J Surg* 103:477, 1962.

74. Engel R: Trauma of the genitourinary system, in Ballinger W, Rutherford R, Zuidema G (eds): *The Management of Trauma* ed 2. Philadelphia, WB Saunders Co, 1973.

75. Guyton A: *Textbook of Medical Physiology*. ed 5, Philadelphia, WB Saunders Co, 1976.

76. Hopson W, Sherman R, Sanders J: Stab wounds of the abdomen. *Am Surg* 32:213, 1966.

77. Jarvis F, Byers W, Platt E: Experiences in the management of the abdominal wounds of warfare. *Surg Gynecol Obstet* 82:174, 1946.

78. Nowak R, Tomlanovich M: Subcutaneous emphysema. *J Amer Coll Emerg Physicians* 6:269, 1977.

79. Backwinkel K: Rupture of the rectus abdominis muscle. *Arch Surg* 90:35, 1965.

80. Carey L, Lowery B, Cloutier C: Hemorrhagic shock. *Curr Prob Surg* January 1971.

81. Olsen W: The serum amylase in blunt abdominal trauma. *J Trauma* 13:200, 1973.

82. Pontes J: Urologic injuries. *Surg Clin N Amer* 56:77, 1977.

83. Adams R, Salam M: Acute and subacute myopathic paralysis, in Thorn G, Adams R, Braunwald E, et al (eds): *Harrison's Principles of Internal Medicine* ed 8. New York, McGraw-Hill, 1977.

84. Cook G, Barkin M, Schillinger J: Urological injuries, in Salter R (ed): *Care for the Injured Child*. Baltimore, Williams and Wilkins Co, 1975, p 166.

85. Love L: Radiology of abdominal trauma. *JAMA* 231:1377, 1975.

86. Olsen W, Hilbreth D: Abdominal paracentesis or peritoneal lavage. *J Trauma* 11:824, 1971.

87. Engrav L, Benjamin C, Strate R, et al: Diagnostic peritoneal lavage in blunt abdominal trauma. *J Trauma* 15:854, 1975.

88. Ahmad W, Polk H: Blunt abdominal trauma. *Arch Surg* 111:489, 1976.

89. Fischer R, Beverlin B, Engrav L, et al: Diagnostic peritoneal lavage. *Am J Surg* 136:701, 1978.

90. Thal E, Shires G: Peritoneal lavage in blunt abdominal trauma. *Am J Surg* 125:64, 1973.

91. McAvoy J, Cook H: A treatment plan for rapid assessment of the patient with massive blood loss and pelvic fracture. *Arch Surg* 113:986, 1978.

92. Thal E: Evaluation of peritoneal lavage and local exploration in lower chest and abdominal stab wounds. *J Trauma* 17:642, 1977.

Fractures and Dislocations

George Sternbach, M.D.
Assistant Medical Director
Emergency Services
Stanford University Medical Center
Stanford, California

FRACTURES AND DISLOCATIONS frequently are dramatic and challenging emergency problems. When present with airway failure or cardiovascular compromise, musculoskeletal injuries assume secondary importance in overall patient management. Respiratory tract management and correction of hypovolemia take precedence in the treatment of the injured patient.

Exsanguinating hemorrhage is the potential consequence of relatively few musculoskeletal injuries. Only fractures of the pelvis and femoral shaft commonly result in hypovolemic shock. Neurovascular injury is a far more frequent complication of fractures and dislocations. Therefore, assessment of motor and sensory function, pulses and capillary filling distal to a musculoskeletal injury are of great importance.

The clinical findings indicative of fracture are tenderness, deformity, swelling, ecchymosis, instability and crepitation. The latter two are the most reliable findings, but the manipulation required to demonstrate them is often intensely painful, as well as potentially injurious to periosseous structures.

Dislocation is accompanied by pain, swelling, deformity and limitation of motion. Capsular, ligamentous and cartilaginous injuries are frequent accompaniments to dislocation and result in joint stiffness, instability and degenerative arthritis, which are its late sequelae. Duration of immobilization following reduction depends upon the joint involved. Upper-extremity joints, which do not serve a weight-bearing function, need be immobilized for a shorter time than those of the lower extremity.[1]

Falls from heights result in more lower-than upper-extremity injuries, with fractures of the calcaneous, tibia, fibula and femur predominating.[2,3] Automobile accidents result in a variety of musculoskeletal trauma, but some injuries are characteristic. In one large series, most posterior fracture-dislocations of the hip were the result of automobile accidents, in which the knee of an unrestrained occupant hit the dashboard.[4] Lower-extremity fractures also predominate in motorcycle accidents, with open, comminuted fractures or segmental bone loss frequently complicating the injuries.[5]

In open fractures, the cutaneous wound may be some distance from the osseous injury—a fact frequently noted in open fractures of the femur. Judicious wound care and the use of antibiotics and tetanus prophylaxis are important. Many of these injuries require operative debridement.

The age of a patient dictates not only the type of injury likely but prognostic and

therapeutic considerations as well. The epiphyses and their perichondral rings constitute the weakest portions of a child's bone and are, therefore, frequently fractured. Epiphyseal plate injuries should be recognized and categorized according to the Salter-Harris classification system.[6] Radiographic findings may be subtle, and such injuries may be misdiagnosed as sprains. Physical examination of a child with ligamentous injury, however, will reveal tenderness along the course of a ligament only, whereas epiphyseal plate fracture will produce tenderness on both sides of the bone. Since ligamentous tissue is generally stronger than growing bone, sprains are less common injuries in children than fractures.[7]

Fractures in children occur more frequently in the upper extremities than the lower.[8] The type and location of injury is likely to be different in the child than the adult. The child's bone is more porous than that of the adult and is therefore more subject to fracture from bending forces. The previously mentioned strength of the ligaments relative to bone frequently results in avulsion fracture at the sites of attachment of musculotendinous units.[7]

A child's fracture will heal more rapidly than the adult's, however. Growth will also tend to correct angular deformity caused by fracture of a long bone. This is not true of rotational deformity, which must be carefully corrected by the physician at the time of reduction.

The aging process results in osteoporosis, or skeletal atrophy, which renders the older skeleton more susceptible to injury. The atrophy is not a uniform process, however, and results in relatively weaker areas in the vertebrae, pelvis, hip and distal radius of the older skeleton.[9] With advancing age, fractures in these locations become more common.

THE HAND

Although no upper-extremity skeletal injuries are likely to prove sufficiently life threatening to warrant priority attention in the multiply injured patient, the functional importance of the hand makes precise correction of deformity imperative. Fractures of the hand are frequently displaced or angulated, and such deformity is maintained by imbalanced musculotendinous action across a fracture site. Finger fractures can generally be manipulated under metacarpal block anesthesia and reduction maintained by a finger splint. Metacarpal fractures and proximal phalanx fractures require immobilization of the wrist as well.[10] When this is done, the wrist should be placed in 15° to 20° of extension, a position which balances the actions of the long flexor and extensor tendons across the carpus.[11]

Deformities resulting from fractures of the hand are rotation, angulation and shortening. Internal fixation is more likely to be required if significant deformity exists. Rotational deformity is best visualized by viewing the ends of the extended fingertips or by having the patient flex the fingers individually. Each flexed finger should point toward the navicular and rest on the thenar eminence; failure to do so indicates a rotational deformity. Shortening is better tolerated in some bones than others. This is true of metacarpals I, II

and V, for example, which allow for more shortening without signifcant impairment of hand function, than do metacarpals III and IV.[10(p1430–1432)]

Fractures are more common in metacarpals IV and V, which are relatively mobile, than in II and III, which are comparatively fixed in position. Fractures of the metacarpal base and transverse fractures of the shaft often display no angulation deformity and require no reduction. This is not the case with oblique or comminuted fractures, which commonly display significant angulation, shortening or displacement and frequently require internal fixation.[10(p1402–1411)]

Fracture of the neck is the most common type of metacarpal fracture. The "boxer's fracture," an injury to the fifth metacarpal in which the head of the bone is displaced palmarward, is an example. Up to 40° of volar angulation is tolerable. Reduction of greater than 40° of angulation is effected by flexing the proximal phalanx and applying dorsally directed pressure to the proximal interphalangeal joint.[12] The hand should then be immobilized for three to four weeks in a short-arm cast with an outrigger splint maintaining the finger in the position of function.

Another common metacarpal fracture is Bennett's fracture of the first metacarpal base. This is really a fracture-dislocation of the metacarpal, as the distal fragment is displaced radially due to the action of the abductor pollicis longus tendon upon it. Internal fixation, performed either percutaneously or by open procedure, is generally required to maintain a reduction of this fracture.

Tuft fractures of the distal phalanx are

122

usually caused by blunt concussive or crushing injury, with accompanying soft-tissue trauma. Debridement, irrigation and closure of the soft-tissue injury and immobilization in a splint for three weeks is treatment of choice.[11(p84)] Although the fractures are often comminuted, no reduction is necessary.

Dislocations of the bones of the hand are common at the interphalangeal and metacarpophalangeal joints. They are generally easily reducible by application of traction and pressure over the displaced bony prominence. Occasionally, a dislocation will not be reducible by closed means. This most frequently occurs in metacarpophalangeal dislocations and is the consequence of the insinuation of joint capsule between the displaced bones. Open reduction is necessary in these cases.[1(p1398)]

THE WRIST

The navicular is the most commonly fractured carpal bone. A more complete discussion of other carpal fractures is to be found elsewhere.[13] The mechanism of injury in navicular fracture is usually a fall on the outstretched hand. Although the same type of fall can result in Colles's fracture of the distal radius, the latter is found predominantly in postmenopausal females, whereas navicular fractures occur most frequently in young adults.[14] About 70% of navicular fractures occur through the middle third or "waist" of the bone.[15] Due to the vascularization of the bone (most of the blood vessels enter the navicular distally) the prognosis for bony union is better for fractures of the distal tubercle and worse for fractures occurring at the waist and more proximally.[16]

Displaced fractures also have a worse prognosis.[13(p1515-1516)]

Physical findings indicative of fracture are tenderness over the anatomical snuff-box and limitation of motion of the wrist in extension and radial deviation. X-rays may be negative because the central roentgen beam frequently does not traverse the plane of the fracture of a hand placed palm down on an x-ray cassette.[17] Special navicular views may be required. As a result of resorption of bone, fracture lines usually become more evident one to two weeks after injury.

The major complication of navicular fractures, other than those of the tubercle, is nonunion. Such a complication is the result of the degree of motion allowed at the fracture site as well as the navicular's poor vascular supply.[17(p830)] Documented fractures should be casted until radiographic signs of bony union appear. Fractures suspected clinically but not demonstrated on x-ray should be casted and x-rayed two weeks later, at which time the fracture line may be evident.

Although differences of opinion exist regarding the optimal method of immobilization, the short-arm thumb spica is the most common technique. Long-arm plaster immobilization, however, is also advocated and touted as promoting rapid union.[16(p42-44)] Navicular fractures are rarely accompanied by injuries to adjacent bones. Although caused by the same mechanism as the Colles's fracture, navicular and distal radius fractures rarely occur simultaneously. Nevertheless, such combined injuries *do* occur, especially in patients who fall from a height on their outstretched hand.[14(p185-188)]

The most common dislocation of the

carpal bones is anterior dislocation of the lunate. The mechanism of injury is forced extension of the wrist.[18] This is also the mechanism of perilunate dislocation, a less common injury, in which the lunate maintains its normal relationship to the radius but the remainder of the carpus is displaced.

Dislocation of the lunate is accompanied by marked swelling and limitation of motion of the wrist. On anteroposterior view, x-rays reveal the lunate appearing triangular rather than its normal quadrilateral shape. In addition, the densities of the carpal bones overlap. Median nerve injury is a common accompaniment, and the dangers of permanent neurological impairment and avascular necrosis of the lunate mandate prompt reduction. This is accomplished by traction on the fingers, extension of the wrist and pressure over the displaced bone.[1(p1397)]

Radiocarpal dislocations often occur with fracture of the distal radius. Internal fixation is required to maintain reduction of this injury.[13(p1529)]

THE FOREARM

The radius and ulna form a ringlike structure in the forearm and, as is the case in other parts of the body where rings of bone are found, multiple fractures are common. When both the radius and ulna are fractured, treatment with open reduction and internal fixation is generally required for adults, but closed reduction and immobilization are usually adequate for most children.[19]

Isolated fractures of the ulna most frequently occur in the distal portion of the bone and are often caused by a direct blow to the forearm. If displacement is absent or slight, immobilization in a long-arm cast results in satisfactory healing in six to seven weeks. Fractures of the proximal portion of the bone and those that are displaced or comminuted heal more slowly.[20]

In 1814, Abraham Colles described the most common, isolated fracture of the radius, a fracture that now bears his name as an eponym. He portrayed in exacting detail the deformity of "a fracture, seated about an inch and a half above the carpal extremity of the radius."[21] This deformity is produced by the dorsal angulation of the distal fragment and is usually amenable to reduction by traction and volarly directed pressure on the distal fragment under local or regional anesthesia. The reduction may be maintained by a long-arm cast. If swelling is severe, a sugar tong splint may be applied.

The reverse Colles or Smith fracture is caused by a fall on the flexed wrist. The radius is fractured in its distal portion, and the distal fragment is displaced in a volar direction. The mechanism of reduction is similar to that of the Colles fracture except that the force of pressure applied to the distal fragment is in a dorsal direction. Precise reduction is essential, and the reduction must frequently be secured with internal fixation.[22] Fracture of the more proximal distal radius with angulation is known as the Piedmont or Galeazzi fracture. A most unstable fracture, it almost invariably requires internal fixation.[22(p164)]

THE ELBOW

Fractures of the olecranon process of the ulna if displaced require excision of the

124 proximal ulna or internal fixation. The mechanism of injury is usually a fall on the point of the elbow.[23] Likewise, fractures of the radial head that are comminuted or involve significant articular surface require resection of the head. Such fractures may be produced by forces transmitted along the radius in falling on the hand and may, in fact, accompany a fracture of the wrist.[24] Fractures involving a minimum of the radial articular surface respond to short-term immobilization in a sling.

Radial head dislocation most commonly occurs with a fracture of the shaft of the ulna, the Monteggia fracture. This fracture is usually treated with open reduction and internal fixation of the ulnar fracture.[24(p388)] Subluxation of the radial head occurs in small children, who typically sustain the injury when an adult forcefully pulls upward on their arm. The child refuses to use the arm, allowing it to dangle at the side. There is resistance to full passive supination as performed by the examiner. X-rays are normal. The injury is caused by the insinuation of torn fibers of the orbicular ligament between the radial head and the capitellum of the humerus. It is reduced by flexing the elbow to 90°, maintaining pressure over the radial head and supinating the forearm.[1(p1395)]

The flexed elbow is dislocated posteriorly by a fall on the outstretched hand. Swelling and deformity of the joint are pronounced. The elbow is extended and cannot be flexed. Reduction is achieved by applying traction to the forearm and countertraction against the humerus. Alternatively, the dislocation can be reduced by applying traction in the direction of the long axis of the dangling forearm.[25]

Following reduction, the elbow, flexed to 90°, is immobilized in a sling and posterior splint. Range of motion exercises should be instituted at an early stage. Although two to three weeks' immobilization is usually advocated, as little as one day of immobilization following dislocation has been reported.[26]

THE ARM

Supracondylar fractures of the humerus in children are rightfully regarded as potentially among the most devastating of bony injuries. The most common childhood fracture about the elbow, it is a cause of radial, median and ulnar nerve injuries. In addition to this, compression, contusion or laceration of the brachial artery may occur, resulting in vascular compromise and Volkmann's ischemia. A thorough neural and circulatory evaluation is essential. This evaluation must extend beyond mere palpation of the radial pulse, because in some instances the peribrachial collateral circulation is sufficient to sustain the arm without radial pulsation.[27]

Closed reduction of the fracture has traditionally been utilized in preference to an open procedure, as the latter has not produced results significantly superior to warrant the risk of surgery.[28] However, surgery is necessary if vascular compromise occurs.

Fracture of the mid to distal shaft of the humerus should suggest possible radial nerve injury. Radial nerve function may be tested by having the patient extend the wrist and metacarpophalangeal joints. Immobilization of such fractures may be achieved with light splints and a sling or with a simple hand sling. A hanging cast may cause distraction of the fragments and thereby delay healing.[29]

Fractures of the neck of the humerus generally do not entail serious complications. The most common immediate complication is brachial plexus injury, caused by trauma to the arm and not the fracture per se. Since reports of axillary artery injury with humeral neck fractures have been cited, attention to the circulation of the arm is warranted.[30]

THE SHOULDER

The shoulder girdle is an intricate complex consisting of seven separate joints. The largest of these, the glenohumeral joint is a shallow ball-and-socket joint with a large natural range of motion. The price paid for this range of motion is relative instability: the glenohumeral joint is frequently dislocated.

Anterior dislocation of the humeral head is more common than posterior. The usual causes are falling on the outstretched arm, forcible external rotation of the arm or backward displacement of the abducted arm.[1(p1394)] Dislocation is common in the young, although it can occur at any age, because in young individuals, the proximal humerus is stronger than the periarticular ligaments. Therefore, given the appropriate degree of trauma, dislocation rather than fracture will occur in many instances.[31]

Examination reveals an abnormal contour of the shoulder, prominence of the angular acromion and marked limitation of motion. X-rays confirm the diagnosis and should be taken prior to reduction to ascertain the coexistence of a fracture. Although brachial plexus injuries occasionally occur with this injury,[32] the most commonly damaged structure is the axillary nerve, which provides sensation to the lateral aspect of the shoulder and motor function to the deltoid.

Reduction may be achieved by traction with countertraction, traction on the dangling arm or the Kocher maneuver. Successful reduction is often predicated upon adequate muscular relaxation. Immobilization in a Valpeau dressing for three weeks should follow reduction. Recurrence of dislocation is a frequent complication.

Posterior dislocation is frequently caused by violent injury, generated, for example, by an epileptic seizure or electrical shock. On examination, the rounded contour of the shoulder is flattened anteriorly. The patient is unable to rotate the arm externally. Anteroposterior x-rays of the shoulder may appear normal, so views in another plane, either axillary or transthoracic, are necessary. Reduction is by traction, internal or external rotation and pressure applied over the humeral head posteriorly.

The acromioclavicular joint is frequently disrupted, even by relatively minor trauma, usually a fall on the point of the shoulder. The joint depends for its stability on the acromioclavicular and coracoclavicular ligaments, the latter being the stronger of the two. Separations are graded according to the degree of injury. Grade I separations involve incomplete injury to the acromioclavicular ligament only. Despite marked swelling and tenderness over the joint and profound pain on attempted abduction of

126 the shoulder, there is no instability and x-rays are normal.

Grade II separation involves tearing of the acromioclavicular ligament. Physical examination reveals the deformity of the distal clavicle displaced superior to the acromion. X-rays confirm the displacement, which is usually less than the width of the clavicle. Weight-bearing films, taken with the patient holding ten-pound weights, may accentuate the displacement.

Grade III separations are the result of rupture of both the acromioclavicular and coracoclavicular ligaments. Deformity is prominent, with the distal clavicle being easily palpable. If ligament rupture is complete, less discomfort is felt upon motion than in Grade I or II separations.

Grade I or II separations require treatment with sling immobilization only. Some difference of opinion exists regarding open versus closed treatment of more severe injuries. Initial treatment for Grade III separations should be a sling, such as the Kenny-Howard sling, which applies the weight of the arm to the distal clavicle, reducing the deformity.[33]

Clavicular fractures, supposedly the most common fractures of the entire body, are most frequently caused by a fall on the outstretched arm or point of the shoulder.[34] Neurovascular complications, although occasionally encountered, are uncommon.[35] Displacement and resulting non-union are encountered most frequently in distal clavicular fractures. Immobilization in a figure-of-eight bandage, the traditional treatment, may exacerbate the displacement of distal clavicular fractures, for which a sling similar to that used for acromioclavicular separation is more appropriate.[36] Even for midclavicular fractures, a full-arm sling may be equally efficacious and is certainly more comfortable than the figure-of-eight bandage.[37]

Unlike the clavicle, the scapula is rarely fractured. A strong, flat bone, it requires considerable force to break. Many scapular fractures are the result of automobile or motorcycle accidents. As they are frequently associated with rib and clavicular fractures, as well as head, intrathoracic and renal injuries, a scapular fracture is warning of the possibility of such injuries.[38]

THE PELVIS

Fractures of the pelvis represent the most dangerous of all bony injuries, as they are capable of causing exsanguinating hemorrhage. The source of such bleeding is usually the vascular plexus lining the pelvic walls and the fractured bones themselves. Occasionally, injured iliac, iliolumbar or femoral vessels contribute to the blood loss.[39,40] Hemorrhage is retroperitoneal, though the retroperitoneal hematoma may rupture into the peritoneal cavity.

When signs of hypovolemic shock are present, early transfusion of blood is mandatory. Reduction of unstable pelvic fractures will also diminish bleeding.[41] Adjunctive measures that reduce hemorrhage and counteract hypovolemia, such as utilization of the antishock suit, may be needed. The suit is particularly useful in retroperitoneal hemorrhage, where isolated bleeding sites amenable to surgical ligation are frequently not present.

Major fractures with which severe

hemorrhage is most often associated are fractures of the sacrum or ilium, bilateral fractures of the pubic rami, separation of the symphysis pubis and dislocations of the sacroiliac joint.[42] Minor fractures, which are stable and can be treated with bed rest followed by gradual weight bearing, are unilateral ischial, pubic ramus and avulsion fractures.[39]

Urinary tract injury accompanies approximately 10% of pelvic fractures. Hematuria is seen in most such injuries but may also be present without significant urologic damage. Injuries to the bladder and urethra occur most commonly with fractures of the pubic rami or separation of the symphysis pubis. Rupture of the bladder occurs most often in the extraperitoneal portion and results in urinary extravasation into the perivesical tissue. Diagnosis is made by retrograde cystography.[39(p104–110)]

In males, urethral injuries frequently occur at the level of the prostatic apex. Tears are complete in most cases. Gross blood is seen at the urethral meatus. Pubic fractures may be palpable on rectal examination. The prostate, displaced superiorly, is surrounded by a boggy collection of blood and urine. Urethrography confirms the diagnosis.[43]

Nerve injuries complicating pelvic fractures are uncommon but are frequently overlooked.[44] Neurological deficit is more likely to accompany fractures of the sacrum than other pelvic injuries. The femoral and sciatic nerves are the structures most frequently subject to injury.[45] The former innervates the extensor muscles of the knee, while the latter supplies the extensors of the great toe. The functions of these muscles should, therefore, be assessed in the patient with a pelvic fracture.

THE HIP

Fractures of the hip occur primarily in elderly individuals. They are rare in children and are associated with a high incidence of avascular necrosis of the femoral capital epiphysis.[46] The leg is typically flexed, externally rotated and shortened. There is severe pain on manipulation of the hip. If the fracture is proximal to the intertrochanteric area, bleeding is slight, and volume replacement is not a critical part of resuscitation.

Dislocations of the hip occur posteriorly ten to 20 times as often as anteriorly.[47] Considerable violence is usually required to cause the injury. Automobile and motorcycle accidents and falls from heights are frequent causes.[48] Posterior dislocations result from forced approximation of the knee and hip. On physical examination, the hip is flexed and adducted; the leg is shortened and internally rotated.

X-rays usually reveal the upward and backward displacement of the femoral head. However, the anteroposterior view of the joint may appear normal, and a lateral view may be required to make the diagnosis. Complications include sciatic nerve injury, avascular necrosis of the femoral head and degenerative arthritis.[49] The latter is more likely if loose fragments of bone or cartilage remain in the joint.[50] Primary open reduction and debridement of such comminuted injuries has been advocated.[4(p1103)] Associated fractures of

128 the femoral head [50] or shaft [48(p254)] occur on occasion, so the entire femur should be examined and x-rays ordered as indicated.

Closed reduction may be accomplished by several methods. With the hip and knee flexed and the patient supine, traction is placed on the femur with countertraction on the pelvis. Some rotation of the femur may be necessary. Alternatively, the patient may be placed prone with the hip hanging over the edge of the examination table. Downward traction with some rotation is then applied on the femur. Due to the powerful muscles of the thigh about the hip, reduction is frequently difficult, and a general anesthetic may be necessary.

THE FEMUR

Fracture of the femur is frequently caused by automobile accidents or other violent trauma and may result in significant hemorrhage into the thigh. This volume deficit should be replaced as indicated. As soon as possible, traction should be instituted via a Hare traction splint if available, or a Thomas splint. Traction is necessitated by the action of the hamstring, quadriceps and adductor muscles, which tend to produce overriding and angulation of the bony fragments.

Neurovascular damage due to femoral fracture is rare, but such a possibility should be considered in distal fractures because of their proximity to the popliteal vessels and the common peroneal nerve.[51] Volkmann's ischemia is a recognized, though uncommon, complication of femoral fracture.[52] Open fractures are common and incur considerable morbidity because soft-tissue wound management is difficult in the highly compartmentalized, muscular thigh.[53]

THE KNEE

Fractures involving the tibial plateau or distal femur generally cause significant swelling and deformity. Hemarthrosis of the knee contributes to the patient's pain and merits prompt evacuation. The patella may be fractured by a direct blow or indirectly through a violent contraction of the quadriceps muscle.[54] Although such a fracture causes considerable swelling, pain and tenderness to palpation are sometimes surprisingly mild. When the fracture is longitudinal and nondisplaced, the leg should be immobilized in a cylinder cast for eight weeks. However, if the fracture is transverse (a configuration prone to delayed fragment separation) or comminuted, surgical fixation should be considered.[55]

Traumatic dislocation of the patella often follows rotational trauma to the knee. The knee is flexed, and the displaced patella is palpable laterally. This dislocation can be reduced by applying medially directed pressure over the lateral side of the patella.

Dislocation of the knee is a serious injury, due to the tremendous force required to disrupt this stable joint. The major morbidity is a result of injury to the popliteal artery. When such injury occurs, circulation to the distal leg is endangered because the fragile genicular arteries are frequently severed as well.[56] The danger of popliteal artery injury is evident from the fact that the amputation rate has not changed significantly for the past 20 years.[57]

The frequent association of vascular injury with knee dislocation, an incidence of around 40%, is explained by the anatomy of the popliteal space.[58] The popliteal artery is bound down at either end of the space by membranous attachments but is strung across the fossa like a bowstring. Disruption of bony anatomical relationships, therefore, disposes the artery to injury.

The dislocation must be reduced as soon as it is diagnosed. With substantial damage to periarticular ligaments, this is readily accomplished by traction and re-alignment of the bones. Distal circulation must be assessed, although the presence of popliteal pulse does not assure that vascular injury has not occurred. Arteriography is indicated in all cases.[57(p780)]

Traction injuries of the peroneal and tibial nerves also occur, but since actual severance of the nerves is uncommon, prognosis for return of neural function is good.[59] Surprisingly, associated injury to other bony structures is rare.[58(p194)]

THE LEG

Forces which break the tibia frequently fracture the fibula as well, athough not necessarily at the same level. Isolated fractures of the fibular shaft do occur, but since the shaft serves no weight-bearing function, such fractures require little attention.[60]

The tibia is susceptible to fracture in a number of ways. During childhood, this bone is a more frequent site of stress fracture than are the metatarsals.[61] Plateau fractures are often incurred in falls and traffic accidents, especially accidents in which a pedestrian is struck by an auto. Fractures of the shaft caused by low-energy impact tend to be either closed transverse or longitudinal. High-energy injuries result in transverse fractures, which are open or comminuted. Serious complications may attend the latter, including wound and bone infection, skin necrosis, delayed union, non-union and venous thrombosis.[62]

The scant amount of soft tissue overlying the tibia anteriorly commonly results in open fractures. Damage to skin, muscle and soft tissue may be considerable, especially in transverse fractures. Delayed fracture healing and wound infection are more likely in high-energy injuries. Antibiotic therapy should be instituted, covering streptococci, staphylococci and also Gram negative organisms.[63] Although one assumes that an open injury invariably prevents compartment compression from developing, this is not necessarily the case. Fragments of torn muscle or fascia may occlude muscular compartments and the expected decompression does not occur.[53(p1441)]

Increased intracompartmental pressure with resulting ischemic necrosis of the contained structures is the most devastating of tibia fracture complications. The anterior compartment contains the tibialis anterior muscle, the anterior tibial vessels and the deep peroneal nerve. Signs of anterior compartment compression are inability to dorsiflex the foot, pain on passive motion of the toes and diminished sensation over the dorsal first web space.

The lateral compartment contains the peroneal muscles, the superficial peroneal nerve and the peroneal vessels. Loss of strength in foot eversion and sensory deficit on the dorsum of the foot indicate a lateral compartment compression. The posterior compartment, containing the soleus and gastrocnemius muscles, is seldom affected by compression following tibial fracture.

Many types of injuries may cause increased intracompartmental pressure, although this is rarely the result of tibial plateau fracture.[64] Since early signs of ischemia may be subtle, intra-fascial pressure is an objective indication for surgery. Pressures in excess of 40 mm Hg indicate that arteriolar pressure has been exceeded[65] and demonstrate the need for fasciotomy.

THE ANKLE AND FOOT

Many fractures of the ankle may be managed by closed reduction and plaster immobilization. Reduction must be along anatomical lines and consider mechanism of injury. The Lauge-Hansen classification of ankle fractures should be utilized.[66]

The fifth metatarsal is the most frequently fractured. The base of this bone is often injured as a result of sudden inversion of the foot. The degree of immobilization required depends upon the discomfort experienced by the patient. The middle metatarsals are subject to stress fracture, which calls for immobiliza-

tion in a short-leg walking cast for three to four weeks.

Fracture of the calcaneus is classically the result of a fall from a height and is the most common of major tarsal injuries.[67] A severe trauma is necessary to fracture the calcaneus and such a fracture is accompanied by spinal column injury in 10% of cases.[68] Other associated injury sites are the soft tissue of the foot, the skin and ligamentous structures. The calcaneal articular surface may be damaged beyond recovery.[69]

Radiographic assessment should include both lateral and axial views—the latter being required to demonstrate the medial and lateral surfaces of the calcaneus.[70]

Controversy surrounds optimal definitive management of calcaneal fractures. Initial care should include cooling and elevation of the foot to reduce the extensive swelling that invariably accompanies this injury. In addition, a search should be made for associated injuries, especially of the spine, whose significance eclipses that of calcaneal fracture.

SUMMARY

Emergency management of fractures and dislocations requires attention not only to bony injury but also to damage to neural, vascular and soft tissue structures. Appropriate treatment requires knowledge of regional anatomy, trauma mechanisms and commonly associated injuries. Prioritization of the bony injuries in the multiply injured patient is of the essence.

REFERENCES

1. Meyers MH: Dislocations: Diagnosis, management and complications. *Surg Clin N Amer* 48:1391–1402, 1958.
2. Reynolds BM, Balsand NA, Reynolds FS: Falls from heights: A surgical experience of 200 consecutive cases. *Ann Surg* 174, 1971.
3. Greenberg MI: Falls from heights. *JACEP* 7:300–301, 1978.
4. Epstein HC: Posterior fracture-dislocations of the hip. *J Bone Joint Surg* 56A:1103–1127, 1974.
5. Haddad JP, et al: Motorcycle accidents: A review of 77 patients treated in a three-month period. *J Trauma* 16:550–557, 1976.
6. Salter RB, Harris R: Injuries involving the epiphyseal plate. *J Bone Joint Surg* 45A:587–622, 1963.
7. Eilert RE: Sports injuries in children. *Surg Rounds* 1:54–62, 1978.
8. Reed MH: Fractures and dislocations of the extremities in children. *J Trauma* 17:351–354, 1977.
9. Chalmers J: Distribution of osteoporotic changes in the aging skeleton. *Clin Endoc Met* 2:203–220, 1973.
10. Brown PW: The management of phalangeal and metacarpal fractures. *Surg Clin N Amer* 53:1393–1437, 1973.
11. Golden GT, et al: Fractures of the phalanges and metacarpals: An analysis of 555 fractures. *JACEP* 6:79–84, 1977.
12. Posner MA: Injuries to the hand and wrist in athletes. *Orth Clin N Amer* 8:593–618, 1977.
13. Dunn AW: Fractures and dislocations of the carpus. *Surg Clin N Amer* 52:1513–1538, 1972.
14. Stother IG: A report of 3 cases of simultaneous Colles' and scaphoid fractures. *Injury* 7:185–188, 1976.
15. Russe O: Fracture of the carpal navicular. *J Bone Joint Surg* 42A:759–768, 1960.
16. Broome A, Cedell CA, Colleen S: High plaster immobilisation for fracture of the carpal scaphoid bone. *Acta Chir Scand* 128:42–44, 1964.
17. Thorndike A Jr, Garrey WE: Fractures of the carpal scaphoid. *N Engl J Med* 222:827–830, 1940.
18. Campbell RD Jr, Lance EM, Yeoh CB: Lunate and perilunar dislocations. *J Bone Joint Surg* 46B:52–72, 1964.
19. Thomas EM, Tuson KWR, Browne PSH: Fractures of the radius and ulna in children. *Injury* 7:120–124, 1975.
20. Altner PC, Hartman JT: Isolated fractures of the ulnar shaft in the adult. *Surg Clin N Amer* 52:155–170, 1972.
21. Colles A: On the fracture of the carpal extremity of the radius. *Edinburgh Med Surg J* 10:182–186, 1814.
22. Cautilli RA, et al: Classifications of fractures of the distal radius. *Clin Orthop Rel Res* 103:163–166, 1974.
23. Newell RML: Olecranon fractures in children. *Injury* 7:33–36, 1975.
24. Grimes HA: Adult elbow injuries. *J Ark Med Soc* 73:388–392, 1977.
25. Meyn MA, Quigley TB: Reduction of posterior dislocation of the elbow by traction on the dangling arm. *Clin Orthop Rel Res* 103:106–108, 1974.
26. Protzman RR: Dislocation of the elbow joint. *J Bone Joint Surg* 60A:539–541, 1978.
27. Lipscomb PR, Burleson RJ: Vascular and neural complications in supracondylar fractures of the humerus in children. *J Bone Joint Surg* 37A:487–492, 1955.
28. Weiland AL, et al: Surgical treatment of displaced supracondylar fractures of the humerus in children. *J Bone Joint Surg* 60A:657–661, 1978.
29. Spak I: Humeral shaft fractures. Treatment with a simple hand sling. *Acta Orthop Scand* 49:234–239, 1978.
30. Theodorides T, de Keizer G: Injuries of the axillary artery caused by fractures of the neck of the humerus. *Injury* 8:120–123, 1976.
31. Neer CS II, Wels RP: The shoulder in sports. *Orthop Clin N Amer* 8:583–591, 1977.
32. McManus F: Brachial plexus lesions complicating anterior fracture-dislocation of the shoulder joint. *Injury* 8:63–66, 1976.
33. Behling F: Treatment of acromioclavicular separations. *Orthop Clin N Amer* 4:747–757, 1973.
34. Sankarankutty M, Turner BW: Fractures of the clavicle. *Injury* 7:101–106, 1975.
35. Yates DW: Complications of fractures of the clavicle. *Injury* 7:189–193, 1976.
36. Allman FL Jr: Fractures and ligamentous injuries of the clavicle and its articulations. *J Bone Joint Surg* 49A:774–784, 1967.
37. Mullick S: Treatment of mid-clavicular fractures. *Lancet* 1:499, 1967.
38. Imatani RJ: Fractures of the scapula: A review of 53 fractures. *J Trauma* 15:473–478, 1975.
39. Conolly WG, Hedberg, EA: Observations on fractures of the pelvis. *J Trauma* 9:104–111, 1969.
40. Patterson FP, Morton KS: The cause of death in fractures of the pelvis. *J Trauma* 13:849–856, 1973.
41. Dunn AW, Morris HD: Fractures and dislocations of the pelvis. *J Bone Joint Surg* 50A:1639–1648, 1968.

132

42. Holm CL: Treatment of pelvic fractures and dislocations. *Clin Orthop Rel Res* 97:97–107, 1973.
43. Morehouse DD, MacKinnon KJ: Urological injuries associated with pelvic fractures. *J Trauma* 9:479–496, 1969.
44. Patterson FP, Morton KS: Neurological complications of fractures and dislocations of the pelvis. *J Trauma* 12:1013–1023, 1972.
45. Goodell CL: Neurological deficits associated with pelvic fractures. *J Neurosurg* 24:837–842, 1966.
46. Weiner DL, O'Dell HW: Fractures of the hip in children. *J Trauma* 9:62–76, 1969.
47. Amihood S: Anterior dislocation of the hip. *Injury* 7:107–110, 1975.
48. Miller CH III, Gustilo R, Tambornino J: Traumatic hip dislocation. *Minn Med* 253–260, 1971.
49. Thompson VP, Epstein HC: Traumatic dislocation of the hip. *J Bone Joint Surg* 33A:746–778, 1951.
50. Chakraborti S, Miller IM: Dislocation of the hip associated with fracture of the femoral head. *Injury* 7:134–142, 1975.
51. Stewart MJ, Sisk TD, Wallace SL: Fractures of the distal third of the femur. *J Bone Joint Surg* 48A:784–807, 1966.
52. Thomson SA, Mahoney LJ: Volkmann's ischemic contracture and its relationship to fracture of the femur. *J Bone Joint Surg* 33B:336–347, 1951.
53. Burkhalter WE: Open injuries of the lower extremity. *Surg Clin N Amer* 53:1439–1457, 1973.
54. Grossman RB, Nicholas JA: Common disorders of the knee. *Orthop Clin N Amer* 8:619–640, 1977.
55. Mitchell WJ: Knee injuries. *Primary Care* 2:383–410, 1975.
56. Lefrak EA: Knee dislocation. *Arch Surg* 111:1021–1024, 1976.

57. O'Donnell TF Jr, et al: Arterial injuries with fractures and/or dislocations of the knee. *J Trauma* 17:775–784, 1977.
58. Shields L, Mital M, Cave EF: Complete dislocations of the knee: Experience at the Massachusetts General Hospital. *J Trauma* 9:192–215, 1969.
59. Reckling FW, Peltier LF: Acute knee dislocations and their complications. *J Trauma* 9:181–191, 1969.
60. Watson-Jones R: The classic: Fractures and joint injuries. *Clin Orthop Rel Res* 105:4–10, 1974.
61. Pilgaard S, Poulsen JO, Christensen JH: Stress fractures. *Acta Orthop Scand* 47:167–169, 1976.
62. Karlstrom G, Olerud S: Fractures of the tibial shaft. *Clin Orthop Rel Res* 105:82–115, 1974.
63. Clancey GJ, Hansen ST: Open fractures of the tibia. *J Bone Joint Surg* 60A:118–122, 1978.
64. Schulak DJ, Gunn DR: Fractures of the tibial plateaus. *Clin Orthop Rel Res* 109:166–177, 1975.
65. Lueck RA, Ray RD: Volkmann's ischemia of the lower extremity. *Surg Clin N Amer* 52:145–153, 1972.
66. Lange-Hansen N: Fractures of the ankle. *Am J Roentgenol* 71:456–471, 1954.
67. Cave EF: Fracture of the os calcis—The problem in general. *Clin Orthop Rel Res* 30:64–66, 1963.
68. Lance EM, Carey EJ Jr, Wade PA: Fractures of the os calcis: Treatment by early mobilization. *Clin Orthop Rel Res* 30:76–89, 1963.
69. Harris RI: Fractures of the os calcis: Treatment by early subtalar arthrodesis. *Clin Orthop Rel Res* 30:100–110, 1963.
70. Aitken AP: Fractures of the os calcis: Treatment by closed reduction. *Clin Orthop Rel Res* 30:67–75, 1963.

Trauma in the Pregnant Patient

Paul S. Auerbach, M.D.
Junior Resident
Department of Emergency Medicine
UCLA Center for the Health Sciences
Los Angeles, California

I N TODAY'S SOCIETY, the pregnant woman does not remove herself from the mainstream of activity and is therefore subject to the same accidental injuries and multiple trauma as her nonpregnant counterpart. Fainting spells, hyperventilation and easy fatigability are common in early pregnancy. These aspects of pregnancy combined with awkwardness from a protuberant abdomen, lordotic posture, and loosening of the pelvic joints, increase the risk of minor accidental trauma.[1,2]

The management of minor accidents poses no special problem for the physician; however, the gravid female who has sustained major injuries must be handled with knowledgeable haste and confidence. The emergency physician must be concerned with the lives of both the mother and fetus, and therefore needs to be familiar with principles of management unique to the pregnant woman. It is the purpose of this discussion to set forth the parameters and principles of treatment and special precautions that must be taken when a pregnant female presents to the emergency department.

134 PATHOPHYSIOLOGY
OF PREGNANCY

Multiple organ systems may be traumatized, and thus it is imperative that the physician understand the natural progression of gestation. Pregnancy represents an alteration in certain physiologic and, to a lesser extent, anatomic considerations.

Of paramount importance to the traumatologist is the fact that during pregnancy blood volume gradually increases approximately 50% over the initial prepregnancy value. The increase in plasma volume exceeds the increase in red cell mass, causing a measurable decrease in hematocrit, from a prepregnancy value of 41.7 to a peripartum value of 37.0.[3] This may alter the usual clinical parameters used to diagnose nonvisible hemorrhage, as significant blood loss may occur (upwards of 30% to 35% of the total blood volume) before hypovolemia becomes manifest by tachycardia or postural hypotension.[4] Additionally, central venous pressure normally decreases during pregnancy to two thirds of the prepregnancy measurement.[5]

The leukocyte count increases from a prepregnancy count of 4,500 cells per cu mm to up to 18,000 cells per cu mm in the last trimester, and 25,000 cells per cu mm during delivery, without any significant change in the differential count.[6,7] This poses a diagnostic problem with infection. An elevated erythrocyte sedimentation rate is similarly of limited value, as it may be elevated normally in pregnancy.

Although serum electrolytes are usually in the normal range, expansion of the extracellular fluid in pregnancy may cause a dilutional hyponatremia, which may be further exacerbated by imposed restrictions in salt intake. The gastrointestinal tract displays an overall hypomotility, with delayed emptying in the stomach and an increase in intestinal transit time.

During pregnancy there is a gradual increase of 30% to 40% in respiratory tidal volume, with no change in vital capacity, indicating a decrease in residual volume. The combination of increased tidal volume and a normal respiratory rate increases respiratory minute volume and creates a compensated respiratory alkalosis, with a decreased carbon dioxide tension in the alveolar blood from 38.5 mm Hg in prepregnancy to 31.3 mm Hg at term, and a corresponding drop in serum bicarbonate from 23.4 mEq per liter to 21.2 mEq per liter.[8]

Anatomical considerations include a significant protrusion of the abdomen, accompanied by an increase and redistribution of the intra-abdominal contents. The diaphragms are elevated, and a compensatory flaring of the ribs is developed in order to keep intrathoracic volume constant. Abdominal musculature becomes lax and offers less protection to the viscera than a tight, unstretched rectus wall.[9] The pregnant uterus increases in size and becomes increasingly vulnerable to injury after the 12th week of gestation, as it extends out of the pelvis. (See Figure 1.)

In certain cases, it shields those intra-abdominal organs it displaces or covers, providing a hydraulic shock absorber, as it were, dissipating force directed through the anterior abdominal wall toward the abdominal organs. During the first trimester the uterus is protected by the bony pelvis, while in the last two trimesters, the

FIGURE 1.   LOCATION AND RELATIVE SIZE OF UTERUS AT DIFFERENT WEEKS OF GESTATION

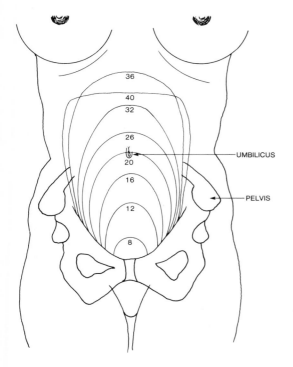

enlarging uterus distends the abdominal wall and at the same time displaces the bowel superiorly. To a certain extent this protects the major blood vessels and intestines from penetrating trauma.[10] The passively stretched abdominal wall in pregnancy may not respond to intraperitoneal irritation, effectively masking the guarding and the rebound tenderness responses, thus rendering the physical examination less reliable.[11]

The supine hypotensive syndrome occurs in pregnant patients as a result of venocaval compression by the enlarged uterine mass. In the supine position, the uterus cuts off venocaval blood flow, pooling blood in the lower extremities, thus diminishing venous return and effectively decreasing cardiac output. This is avoided by placing the patient in a lateral position.

Venous distensibility is increased during pregnancy, and along with venocaval compression accounts for the propensity to varicosity, stasis and vascular trauma. There is an increased vascularity about the uterus, which becomes more prone to hemorrhage upon impact or laceration.

BLUNT TRAUMA DURING PREGNANCY

The kinds of trauma occurring in pregnancy are protean, with accidents estimated to occur in 6.9% of all pregnancies.[12] Far and away the greatest source of trauma is the automobile. In California, it has been estimated that 13.9% of maternal deaths are auto fatalities.[13] High-speed collisions cause a broad spectrum of catastrophic injuries, most often blunt trauma. Apparently, pregnant women are no more prone to vehicular incidents than their non-pregnant counterparts, but the consequences of such incidents are certainly more distressing. The injury varies according to the severity of impact, the seating position of the victim, the type of collision, the size of vehicle and the use of seat belts.[14] The use of seat belts in pregnancy has been controversial; however, properly worn they are of significant benefit. Lap belt restraint decreases the number and severity of injuries resulting from automobile collisions.[15] However, in the pregnant female, the lap belt causes uterine compression and distortion, which may cause shearing of the placental attachments.[16]

136   Sudden deceleration has also, in isolated instances, been associated with mesenteric lacerations, transection of the rectus muscles and bowel, traumatic thrombosis of the mesenteric vessels and abrupt separation of the placenta in the seat-belt wearer.[17] Still, such risks do not outweigh the risks of ejection, head injury and/or chest trauma so commonly the fate of the unrestrained passenger. The seat belt should be worn snugly, well below the dome of the uterus to fit across the pelvis, with a shoulder harness in addition.[18]

Injuries to pregnant victims of automobile collisions tend to be multiple. Indeed, any organ may be injured. Fractures of the pelvis, ribs and skull are common, often complicated by severe soft-tissue injury and hemorrhage.[19] Most maternal deaths are due to head and/or chest injury, whereas fetal death is a result of maternal shock, uterine-placental trauma or direct fetal injury.[20] Less often fatal, but of frequent morbidity, are accidents involving blunt abdominal injury only. The uterus, spleen, kidney, liver and intestines are injured foremost, with injury to the abdominal wall, broad ligament, mesentery, pancreas, diaphragm or retroperitoneum occurring at a much lower frequency.[21, 22] Solid organs are more often injured than hollow viscera, as the latter can deform and better dissipate disruptive forces.

CLINICAL ASPECTS OF BLUNT TRAUMA

Abdominal wall injury is characterized by muscular guarding and rigidity and may present in a fashion similar to intraperitoneal injury. A rectus abdominis hematoma presents as a mass below the umbilicus in over 80% of cases. The hematoma may be distinguished from an intraperitoneal mass by having the patient tighten the abdominal musculature, whereupon the hematoma will remain palpable, while an interabdominal mass disappears. An equivocal examination requires further delineation up to and including laparotomy if necessary.[23]

Rupture of the muscular nonpregnant intrapelvic uterus by external trauma is unusual. However, the pregnant uterus, enlarging into the abdominal cavity, loses the usual bony protection of the pelvis.[24] Rupture of the gravid uterus classically presents with sudden shearing abdominal pain, cessation of uterine contractions, loss of fetal movement and heart tones, vaginal bleeding, hypotension and tachycardia. A previous uterine scar, most often from cesarean section, is often the site of the tear.[25] In the previously nonsurgical uterus, the posterior wall of the fundus is most likely to separate.[26]

Although the injury is major, the symptoms may be no more dramatic than suprapubic pain or diaphragmatic irritation from intraperitoneal blood. Laboratory data are of little value early on. Because of the expanded blood volume in pregnancy, shock may be delayed in onset. Hematuria is commonly associated with isolated urinary tract injury, but may accompany extrusion of the fetus into the bladder. The roentgenographic criteria for rupture of the gravid uterus include a well-defined mass in the abdominal cavity which suggests a contracted uterus, abnormal fetal position outside the confines of the mass, extended fetal extremities, and/or free intraperitoneal air.[27, 28] The index of suspicion must be high, and prompt diagnosis is imperative.

Culdocentesis and peritoneal lavage are useful in the evaluation of intra-abdominal bleeding.

If uterine rupture or transection is recognized, or is highly suspected, surgical intervention is indicated, as infant mortality approaches 100% and maternal exsanguination can be rapid.[29, 30] Procrastination is intolerable, and attempts at medical management may result in death.[31–33] Even though the patient may be in hypovolemic shock, urgent laparotomy is necessary to control hemorrhage, since the shock is secondary to the bleeding.

Traumatic premature separation of the placenta is a rare and serious sequel to blunt trauma, secondary to the shearing of attachments from the inelastic placenta to the readily expansile uterus.[34, 35] Bleeding of variable degrees occurs into the decidua. If less than 25% of the placenta is involved, external vaginal bleeding and premature labor ensue. Greater involvement threatens fetal survival, and greater than 50% separation portends fetal death, accompanied by maternal shock, uterine tetany and possible disseminated intravascular coagulation.[36] Similarly, abruptio placentae can also occur with shock from other causes and may be seen following compression of the inferior vena cava, thus the admonition to avoid the supine recumbent position when the lateral position will do.[37, 38] If abruptio placentae has occurred, fetal distress or labor will ensue, and cesarean section must be rapidly performed. Abruptio placentae should be

suspected whenever there is bleeding from the vagina following trauma.

Blunt trauma may injure the adnexae and result in hemorrhage from disruption of the ovarian or ascending uterine arteries. Torsion of the ovaries may be exquisitely painful and usually presents as a rapidly expanding adnexal mass noted in serial pelvic examinations. Surgical intervention is indicated.

Splenic rupture is the most common intraperitoneal injury due to blunt abdominal trauma, and it is most frequently caused by automobile accidents. Data suggest that pregnancy does not increase the risk of splenic rupture, although one author suggests that distention, displacement and compression of the spleen and liver during pregnancy make them more susceptible to rupture during the third trimester.[39]

The symptoms of splenic rupture are essentially the same in pregnant and nonpregnant patients: left upper quadrant pain, referred pain to the left shoulder (Kehr's sign), nausea, vomiting and leukocytosis to 18,500 cells per cu mm. (This finding, however, is of limited value in pregnancy.) Less frequent indices are left-flank dullness (Ballance's sign) and left-sternocleidomastoid posterior-edge tenderness (Saegesser's sign). Roentgenographic changes include free fluid in the left flank and paracolonic gutter, gastric dilatation with a serrated greater curvature, obliteration of the left psoas and renal shadows and elevations of the left hemidiaphragm. The diagnosis should be a primary consideration in the evaluation of blunt abdominal trauma. Culdocentesis or peritoneal lavage is often necessary and

138

always justified if splenic rupture must be ruled out. The treatment is laparotomy and splenectomy.

Rupture of the diaphragm and resultant diaphragmatic hernia is extremely uncommon. It is manifested by bowel sounds heard over the affected hemithorax, often accompanied by abdominal pain, nausea, emesis, dyspnea, possible cyanosis and shock.[40-42] Roentgenographic changes include extraneous densities in the chest, a mediastinal shift away from the affected hemithorax and atelectasis above an abnormally elevated diaphragm.[43] When the diagnosis is made, surgery is indicated.

Urologic injury as a result of blunt trauma poses no special diagnostic or therapeutic challenge. It is interesting to note that uterine rupture constitutes one of the important causes of bladder injury. Following uterine rupture, the most common signs of concomitant bladder damage are hematuria and meconium-stained urine.[44] Injury to the lower urinary tract occurs in 10% to 15% of cases of pelvic fracture, most commonly with fractures of the pubic rami.[45-48] The female urethra is short and less likely to be transected than the male urethra; however, one such case has been reported.[49]

Usually, pressure on the bladder from blunt trauma will cause it to empty spontaneously. If, however, the force is direct and the anatomic confines of the uterus and symphysis limit decompression, the bladder may burst. The diagnostic studies are no different for the pregnant or nonpregnant patient. Urethral catheterization, cystogram, IVP and cystoscopy are performed, when appropriate. It should be noted that a dilated ureter on the right is often seen in pregnancy as a result of partial obstruction by the uterus and progestational effect. Acute urography is indicated in the delineation of renal trauma in pregnancy, particularly in evaluating the kidney on the contralateral side, when nephrectomy is contemplated.[50] Perirenal extravasation generally indicates a ruptured kidney or structural damage necessitating repair.[51]

Vulvar hematomas result from direct trauma to the perineum and may cause excruciating pain. After careful delineation by pelvic examination, rapidly expanding lesions or those greater than 5 cm require incision and the evacuation of clot. Bleeding vessels should be ligated if visible. More frequently, no distinct bleeders are located and hemorrhage can be controlled with peripheral figure-of-8 sutures, followed by tight packing of the cavity over Penrose drains.

Lacerations of the perineum should be cleansed, debrided and sutured primarily if possible. Rectovaginal tears are closed essentially as episiotomies. Great care must be taken to thoroughly evaluate any vaginal, urethral, rectal or bladder disruptions for more serious injury prior to attempted repair.

In general, skeletal trauma is handled in pregnancy as it is out of pregnancy, with fractures being set primarily and surgical procedures performed. Reports of impairment of fracture healing and altered calcium metabolism in pregnancy have been discussed in the medical literature, but universal agreement does not exist. The trend is to favor internal fixation of fractures over prolonged traction to reduce periods of immobilization, decrease calcium excretion and lessen the risk of thromboembolic disease. Vertebral fractures involving the cervical spine are treated with the usual urgency and respect. Vaginal delivery should not be attempted if there is any chance that the spinal cord may be involved. However, if the spinal cord is acutely involved, there need not be a rush to cesarean section on that account alone. In the absence of other complications, normal pregnancy and labor may follow.[52]

Pelvic fractures in pregnancy are the result of an increase in vehicular accidents and the physiologic relaxation of the pelvic ligaments. Usually these fractures are secondary to pelvic compression, but they may occur from a fall on the heels with resultant calcaneal-vertebral transmission of disruptive forces. The pelvis is a rigid bony ring, and applied forces of from 400 to 2600 pounds are required to disrupt it.[53, 54] Displacement most often occurs in two places because of the ring structure, and usually results in fracture of the pubic and ischial rami from anteroposterior force. This can result in a pelvic outlet obstruction, while lateral crush injuries can cause pelvic inlet obstruction.

A dreaded complication of pelvic fracture is retroperitoneal hematoma, directly related to the increased vascularity of the pelvis in pregnancy and the violent force of the injury. Significant hypovolemia and shock can ensue, as the retroperitoneal space rapidly accumulates up to four liters of blood at pelvic vein pressures.[55] There is some debate about whether pelvic hematomas should be explored. Those who favor surgery point to the necessity of ligation of ruptured or feeding vessels; those who oppose it emphasize retroperitoneal tamponade to control blood loss. What is clear is that fluid resuscitation must be vigorous and immediate to avoid catastrophic fetal and maternal hypotension.

PENETRATING TRAUMA IN PREGNANCY

Penetrating abdominal trauma represents another violent intrusion upon maternal/fetal homeostasis. Although not as common as blunt trauma, fetal injuries have resulted from multitudinous penetrating instruments and missiles, including shrapnel, knives, animal horns, pitchforks, scythes, sickles and (in direct proportion to the recent rise in violent crime) bullets.[56] The uterine wall, amniotic membrane, placenta, umbilical cord and fetus may all be injured. Gunshot wounds are most common in the third trimester, and the morbidity is proportional to the number of organs involved. Those organs that occupy the most space are at greatest risk; thus the gravid uterus, which displaces the small bowel into the upper abdomen and shields other abdominal viscera, is more frequently injured and absorbs most of the energy from a bullet or knife. Indeed, it is rare to have a gunshot wound to the abdomen in the third trimester without uterine involvement.

Still, no maternal deaths from gunshot wounds of the pregnant uterus alone have been reported since 1912.[57] Although the maternal prognosis in gunshot wounds to the uterus is excellent, the fetal outlook is grim. It is generally agreed that high

140 velocity gunshot wounds of the gravid abdomen require prompt operative exploration.[58, 59] This is less emphatically the case with knife and low velocity bullet wounds, because of a lower incidence of multiple injury and more minor wounds.[60] However, if there is any indication of fetal trauma or if the extent of intra-abdominal injury cannot be adequately evaluated, laparotomy is indicated. Stab wounds outside of the abdomen are treated in the traditional fashion. There is a report of a knife laceration of the heart in a pregnant woman, complicated by shock and tamponade, with successful surgical intervention and continuation of pregnancy.[61] There is absolutely no justification for probing any entry tract or attempting to visualize it with radio-opaque contrast material. Both are at the least time consuming and at the worst intrusive and dangerous.

TRAUMA FROM BURNS, ELECTROCUTION AND LIGHTNING

Less common injuries include burns, electrocution and lightning catastrophies. A study of thermal injury in pregnancy has shown that pregnancy does not alter the maternal outcome after major body burns and that fetal survival usually accompanies maternal survival. Following thermal injury, interruption of pregnancy should only be attempted if hypotension, hypoxia or sepsis result in fetal distress.[62, 63] Burn care for the pregnant female requires diligent fluid replacement and vigorous respiratory support to avoid the maternal hypotension and hypoxia that devastate uterine perfusion.

Electrocution causes death by massive current discharge through the body. At least one successful postmortem cesarean section has been reported following this unfortunate event.[64] Conversely, electrical shock of a woman has been reported to cause intrauterine death of her fetus, perhaps on an arrhythmigenic basis.[65]

Lightning injury is a rare event, and even more unusual in the pregnant female. Nonetheless, several cases have been reported, some with successful continuation of the pregnancy.[66] The successful resuscitation of the lightning injured is a function of prompt respiratory support, management of primary ventricular arrhythmias, careful fluid management to avert shock, dilute myoglobin in the urine and prevent renal shut-down, proper tetanus prophylaxis, and thermal burn management.

FETAL INJURY

Fetal injury requires rapid evaluation. In early pregnancy the fetus is protected by the bony pelvis and the amniotic fluid.[67, 68] However, later in pregnancy, the fetal head is stationary within the pelvis, and the amniotic fluid becomes less of a shock absorber. In blunt trauma, intrauterine injuries are most often fractures, usually of the clavicle, leg and skull, although femur, humerus, cervical spine, jaw, rib and tibia fractures have been reported.[69] Skull fractures are most commonly the result of pressure against the maternal pubic symphysis or sacral promontory and usually involve the parietal bones.[70-72] Other injuries may include a ruptured or lacerated spleen, hemoperitoneum, intracranial hemorrhage, contusions of the liver and kidney, adrenal hemorrhage or myocardial contusion.[73-76] Penetrating wounds are more varied, with the potential for the severance and destruction of anything in the path of the intruder. Bullets may perforate the lungs, colon, diaphragm, small bowel and have even been found in the thymus.[77, 78] In one spectacular example, the infant apparently swallowed the bullet in utero and subsequently passed it per rectum after birth.[79]

Fetal mortality is related to fetal maturity, the nature of the wound and the rapidity of treatment. Prematurity is a key negative factor in survival statistics.[80] After the 28th week of gestation, fetal survival has been estimated to be 50%.[81]

EVALUATION OF THE FETUS

The first response of the examining physician should be to record the condition of the fetus. Fetal movement, uterine height and irritability, abdominal tenderness, leakage of amniotic fluid, vaginal bleeding and fetal heart rate must be monitored frequently and accurately from the moment the mother presents to the emergency department.[82] External fetal monitoring transducers should be placed immediately and if labor is imminent, internal fetal scalp electrodes or an intrauterine pressure recorder may be indicated.

Fetal bradycardia less than 110 is the earliest and foremost sign of distress in the fetus that can be saved and points to acute blood loss, decreased uterine blood flow and fetal hypoxia.[83] Fetal scalp blood may be sampled for pH determination; a value less than 7.2 indicates distress. Properly performed, amniocentesis is a useful procedure and may demonstrate meconium or blood in the amniotic fluid. Fetal maturity is indicated by an amniotic fluid creatinine concentration of greater than 1.75 mg % or a lecithin-sphingomyelin ratio of less than 2.0. It should be emphasized that this type of laboratory testing may be a luxury and implies that six to eight hours can be spared prior to intervention.

The indications for cesarean section are essentially the following: if the pregnant uterus prohibits adequate surgical exploration of the injured abdomen, documented abruptio placentae or significant uterine rupture, uncontrollable hemorrhage or other maternal injury resulting in persistent fetal distress, intrauterine infection or death of the mother.

The prematurity of the infant may represent a greater risk to survival than the injuries incurred. A good rule is to interrupt pregnancy only if the fetus is mature and is in distress. Infants less than 1000 g or younger than 30 weeks have little hope of survival, and if at all possible, even in the face of uterine laceration, should be left in utero.[84] This must be balanced against a strong suspicion of serious fetal trauma, in which case the surgeon's hand is forced, and cesarean section must be performed to inspect and treat the infant as best possible.

Maternal death leads directly to fetal death as a result of hypoperfusion of the placenta. However, successful postmortem cesarean section and even vaginal deliveries have been reported. In the event of sudden maternal death, swift cesarean section, preferably within five minutes, should be attempted if there is to be any

142

hope of saving the fetus. On the other hand, fetal death alone does not warrant laparotomy and cesarean section, as the natural course of events will induce a spontaneous miscarriage.

If pregnancy continues normally for several weeks following trauma, subsequent abortion or premature labor is probably not due to the injury. To establish a causal relationship, a normally developed fetus must be aborted within hours of the implicated trauma. Even then, a temporal relationship does not always imply cause.[85] This has important medical and legal implications, for contrary to popular belief, abortion uncommonly follows trauma, unless the fetus dies or there is significant placental disruption.

If the trauma does not terminate the pregnancy, but precipitates premature labor, premature contractions must be stopped. This may be done with strict bed rest and a variety of pharmacotherapeutic interventions. If a possible transient decrease in blood pressure can be tolerated, Diazoxide, a nonthiazide diuretic and arteriolar dilator, can be administered in a single rapid intravenous bolus of 300 mg.[86] Alternatively, an intravenous infusion of 4 g of magnesium sulfate (40 mm of a 10% solution) may be infused slowly, followed by an infusion of 2 g per hour in a 2% solution until the contractions cease or labor is irreversible. If the contractions cease, the infusion is followed by a 1% infusion at 1 g per hour for an additional 24 hours. Contraindications to this method include renal failure or cervical dilatation beyond 5 cm.[87] Alcohol infusions are less effective, and beta-2 sympathomimetics are not yet approved for tocolytic use in the United States.

EVALUATION OF THE PREGNANT PATIENT

Evaluation of the pregnant patient properly begins in the prehospital setting and above all demands the rapid stabilization and transport of the injured to a well-equipped emergency department. In the absence of head trauma critical enough to contraindicate fluid replacement, there must be the immediate initiation of vigorous intravenous crystalloid administration and prompt provision for high-flow oxygen therapy. Cardiac arrhythmias which might compromise maternal and placental perfusion must be swiftly abolished. If significant hypotension is in evidence or imminent, the legs of a properly applied Military Anti-Shock Trousers (MAST) suit may be inflated. Of course, at all times the airway and cervical spine must be protected.

Once the patient arrives in the emergency department, there is absolutely no substitute for a thorough history and physical examination, which should include a pelvic and rectal examination. It is essential to consider the possibility of pregnancy in the initial evaluation of any young woman. The patient should be disrobed and vital signs, both maternal and fetal, monitored regularly and precisely. If the initial evaluation of the patient does not demonstrate vaginal bleeding, uterine irritability, abdominal tenderness, hypovolemia, amniotic fluid leakage or fetal distress, and the patient would not otherwise be admitted, she should be observed for several hours for any change before being discharged.[88]

If hypotension occurs, the patient may be turned to her side or have the legs elevated. The patient should be kept on her side if not contraindicated by other injuries to avoid the hypotension of venocaval compression and excessive pelvic and lower extremity hemorrhage.[89] Airway management is a first and foremost concern, as are head and neck injuries, chest injuries, fractures and dislocations. One, and preferably two, short large-bore intravenous lines should be started immediately to rapidly administer crystalloid, colloid and blood components as necessary to support blood pressure and oxygenation. Up to 35% of maternal blood volume may be lost before hypotension becomes evident. Thus by the time tachycardia and systolic hypotension are apparent, the mother may be near intractable shock. Normotension in the mother is maintained at the expense of the fetal circulation, and the fetus may rapidly become a victim of hypoxia, bradycardia and hypotension, even with only mild maternal hypovolemia.[90]

Maternal blood pressure does not accurately monitor uterine blood flow, as the latter may be reduced by 20% following a major bleed, without changing maternal blood pressure. Catecholamines circulated by the mother in response to shock may cause additional decrements in uterine perfusion while elevating maternal blood pressure. Type-specific whole blood or packed red cells should be used to replace blood losses, for colloids do not improve fetal arterial oxygenation. Until blood can be administered, vigorous infusion of a solution of lactated Ringer's is the fluid replacement of choice.[91,92] Central venous monitoring should be used whenever appropriate. Unless absolutely necessary, vasopressors should not be used, as they decrease uterine blood flow and increase fetal hypoxia.

Tetanus toxoid and tetanus hyperimmune globulin should be administered as they would be in the nonpregnant patient. A nasogastric tube should be placed to prevent vomiting and aspiration in the face of the hypomotility of combined pregnancy and trauma. A sterile Foley catheter should be introduced, if not impeded by a urethral injury, to monitor urinary output and to empty the bladder so that a proper pelvic examination may be performed.

Radiography should be performed as necessary for the proper evaluation of trauma, shielding the fetus where possible and avoiding the unnecessary duplication of films.[93] At all times, the life of the mother should take priority. If there is a reasonable medical indication for the study, the benefits generally outweigh the risks.[94,95]

Blood should be drawn immediately for determination of hemoglobin, hematocrit, white blood count and differential, cross matching, BUN, creatinine, glucose and amylase. Additional blood should be obtained to quantitate SGOT, SGPT, alkaline phosphatase, LDH, calcium, prothrombin time, partial thromboplastin time, platelet count, fibrinogen, fibrin split products, thrombin time and protamine precipitation test. Clotting studies are indicated in the eventuation of disseminated intravascular coagulation. Factors 2, 5, 8 and 10 are classically low.[96] Fibrinogen levels in late pregnancy are normally elevated significantly over prepregnancy levels, so that a "normal" level at term may reflect a severe deficit.

Injury to the placenta, which contains large amounts of thromboplastin, or to the

144 uterus, which contains plasminogen, can induce hypofibrinogenemia due to intravascular consumption coagulopathy.[97,98] Amniotic fluid or meconium embolism is often complicated by intravascular coagulation in patients who survive the initial period of shock and respiratory insufficiency.[99] In such a case, the fetus must be removed and the institution of heparin, which does not cross the placenta, and administration of necessary blood products, platelets and clotting factors must be prompt and vigorous. Post-traumatic pulmonary insufficiency and significant hypoxemia are correlated closely with trauma-induced disseminated intravascular coagulation and may require artificial ventilation.[100]

Peritoneal lavage has been lauded repeatedly for its contribution to the delineation of intra-abdominal trauma, particularly because such injuries often are undiagnosed initially, and delay in diagnosis increases morbidity and mortality.[101] It has been estimated that undiagnosed abdominal injuries are responsible for 12% of deaths from abdominal trauma.[102] This takes on particular significance in the pregnant female, who may not fully manifest the signs of peritoneal irritation or hypovolemia, while the fetus suffers early anoxia as uterine blood flow decreases.[103]

The indications for peritoneal lavage following blunt trauma are abdominal signs and/or symptoms, especially with altered sensorium, unexplained shock, major thoracic injuries and serial changes in hematocrit.[104] The technique is the same for pregnant women and nonpregnant women. After the bladder is emptied and the abdomen prepped, a small horizontal or vertical infraumbilical incision is made under local anesthesia and the tissue dissected down to the peritoneum. A peritoneal dialysis or peritoneal lavage catheter is advanced using a twisting motion through the directly visualized peritoneum and directed toward the pelvis. At this point, if 10 mm of frank blood can be aspirated, the tap is positive. If the aspiration is unrewarding, a liter of lactated Ringer's or normal saline is run wide open into the abdomen and then recovered by gravity. If the lavage fluid is not grossly bloody, a sample should be sent for red cell count, white cell count and amylase. A clearly positive lavage yields one of the following: red blood cell count greater than 100,000 per cu cm, white cell count greater than 500 per cu cm or amylase greater than 175 mg per dl. An alternative to peritoneal lavage is culdocentesis, which may be performed on any female whose other injuries do not preclude this approach to the cul-de-sac.

SUMMARY

The pregnant female imposes a unique challenge and responsibility to the emergency clinician. The emergency physician, surgeon, gynecologist and pediatrician should join forces and blend their skills to preserve the lives of the mother-to-be and her child.

REFERENCES

1. Crosby W: Trauma during pregnancy: maternal and fetal injury. *Obst Gyn Survey* 29:683–699, 1974.
2. Fort AJ, Harlin RS: Pregnancy outcome after non-catastrophic maternal trauma during pregnancy. *Obst Gyn* 35:912–915, June 1970.
3. Quilligan EJ, Kaiser IH: Maternal physiology in Danforth, DN (ed): *Textbook of Obstetrics and Gynecology*. New York, Harper and Row, 1971, pp 231–244.
4. Buchsbaum HJ: Traumatic injury in pregnancy, in Barber HRK, Garber EA: *Surgical Disease in Pregnancy*. Philadelphia, WB Saunders Co, 1974, p 1840.
5. Colditz RJ, Josey WE: Central venous pressure in supine position during normal pregnancy. Comparative determinations during the second and third trimesters. *Obst Gyn* 36:769–772, November 1970.
6. Hakanson EY: Trauma to the female genitalia. *Lancet* 86:287, June 1966.
7. Efrati, et al: Leukocytes of normal pregnant women. *Obst Gyn* 23:429, March 1974.
8. Quilligan EJ, Kaiser IH: Maternal physiology, in Danforth, DN (ed): *Textbook of Obstetrics and Gynecology*. New York, Harper and Row, 1971, pp 231–244.
9. Dyer I, Barclays DL: Accidental trauma complicating pregnancy and delivery. *Am J Obst Gyn* 83:907–929, April 1962.
10. Delaney J: Obstetrical and gynecological injuries, in Ballinger WF, et al (eds): *The Management of Trauma*. Philadelphia, WB Saunders Co, 1973, pp 479–495.
11. Buchsbaum HJ: Accidental injury complicating pregnancy. *Am J Obst Gyn* 102:752–769, November 1968.
12. Peckham CH, King RW: A study of intercurrent conditions observed during pregnancy. *Am J Obst Gyn* 87:609–624, November 1963.
13. Montgomery TA, et al: Maternal deaths in California, 1957–1962. *Calif Med* 100:412–421, June 1964.
14. Raney EH: Fetal death secondary to nonpenetrating trauma of gravid uterus. Paper presented before District 6 meeting of the American College of Obstetrics and Gynecology, Omaha, Nebraska, October 12–15, 1966.
15. Huelke DF, Gikas PW: Causes of death in automobile accidents. *JAMA* 203:1100–1107, March 1968.
16. Crosby W, Costiloe JP: Safety of lap-belt restraint for pregnant victims of automobile collisions. *N Engl J Med* 284:632–636, March 1971.
17. Doersch KB, Dozier WE: The seat belt syndrome. The seat belt sign, intestinal and mesenteric injuries. *Am J Surg* 116:831–833, December 1968.
18. Handel CK: Case report of uterine rupture after an automobile accident. *J Reprod Med* 20:90–92, February 1978.
19. Elliott M: Vehicular accidents and pregnancy. *Aust N Zeal J Obst Gyn* 6:279–286, December 1966.
20. Pepperell RJ, et al: Motor-car accidents during pregnancy. *Med J Aust* 1:203–205, February 1977.
21. Griswold RA, Collier HW: Blunt abdominal trauma. *Internal Abst Surg* 112:309–329, April 1961.
22. Mussalli NG: Uterine, fetal and placental injuries due to a motor car accident. *J Obst Gyn Brit Comm* 79:379–380, April 1972.
23. Shires GT: Trauma in Schwartz SI (ed): *Principles of Surgery*. New York, McGraw-Hill, 1974, pp 195–251.
24. Weinstein EC, Pallais V: Rupture of the pregnant uterus from blunt trauma. *J Trauma* 8:1111–1113, November 1968.
25. Schrinsky DC, Benson RC: Rupture of the pregnant uterus: A review. *Obst Gyn Survey* 33:217–232, April 1978.
26. Dyer T, Barclay R: Accidental trauma complicating pregnancy and delivery. *Am J Obst Gyn* 83:907–929, April 1962.
27. Davidson CN: Roentgen demonstration of fetal death and uterine rupture. *Am J Roentgenol* 62:837–842, December 1949.
28. Mylks GW, et al: X-ray and rupture of the uterus. *Canad Med Ass J* 57:337–340, October 1947.
29. Anteby S, et al: Accidental rupture of the pregnant uterus. *Int Surg* 58:267–268, April 1973.
30. Wilson JR, et al: *Obstetrics and Gynecology*. St. Louis, CV Mosby Co, 1963, p 540.
31. Jacobs WM, et al: Third trimester rupture of the pregnant uterus: A four year study. *Obst Gyn* 19:16–21, January 1962.
32. Keifer WS: Rupture of the uterus. *Am J Obst Gyn* 89:335–348, June 1964.
33. Mathews RI: Rupture of the uterus during pregnancy: A study of 111 cases. *Obst Gyn* 17:551–555, May 1961.
34. Punnonen R: Traumatic premature separation of the placenta. *Annales Chirurgiae et Gynaecologiae Fenniae* 63:487–488, 1974.
35. Peyser MR, Toaff R: Traumatic rupture of the placenta. *Obst Gyn* 34:561–563, October 1969.
36. Page EW, et al: Abruptio placentae: dangers of

146

delay in delivery. *Obst Gyn* 3:385–393, April 1954.

37. Howard BK, Goodson JH: Experimental placental abruption. *Obst Gyn* 2:442, November 1953.

38. Menqert WF, et al: Observations on the pathogenesis of premature separation of the normally implanted placenta. *Am J Obst Gyn* 66:1104–1112, 1953.

39. Buchsbaum JH: Splenic rupture in pregnancy. Report of a case and review of the literature. *Obst Gyn Survey* 22:381–395, June 1967.

40. Bernhardt LC, Lawton BR: Pregnancy complicated by traumatic rupture of the diaphragm. *Am J Surg* 112:918–922, December 1966.

41. Journey RW, Payne RL: Nonobstetric surgical complications during obstetric care: A review of the recent literature. *Am J Med Sci* 232:695–718, December 1956.

42. Carter BN, Giuseffi J: Strangulated diaphragmatic hernia. *Ann Surg* 128:210, 225, August 1948.

43. Carter BN, et al: Traumatic diaphragmatic hernia. *Am J Roentgenol* 65:56–72, January 1951.

44. Raghavaiah NV, Devi AI: Bladder injury associated with rupture of the uterus. *Obst Gyn* 46:573–576, November 1975.

45. Prather GC, Kaiser TF: Bladder in fracture of bony pelvis: Significance of "tear drop bladder" as shown by cystogram. *J Urol* 63:1019–1030, June 1950.

46. Hauser CW, Petry JF: Control of massive hemorrhage from pelvic fractures by hypo-gastric artery ligation. *Surg Gyn Obst* 121:313–315, August 1965.

47. Peltier LF: Complications associated with fractures of the pelvis. *J Bone Joint Surg* 47A:1060–1069, July 1965.

48. Levine JI, Crampton RS: Major abdominal injuries associated with pelvic fractures. *Surg Gyn Obst* 116:223, February 1963.

49. Shah NN, Shah HN: Accidental avulsion of the female urethra. *J Indian Med Ass* 52:434, May 1969.

50. McLean RDW, et al: Acute urography: A method for general use. *Brit Med J* 1:142–144, January 1969.

51. Nunn IN: The management of closed renal injury. *Aust N Zeal J Surg* 31:263–274, May 1962.

52. Comarr AE: Interesting observations on females with spinal cord injury. *Med Services J Canada* 22:651–661, July-August 1966.

53. Chalk PAF, Ford CG: Gross traumatic disruption of the pelvic ring in pregnancy. *J Obst Gyn Brit Comm* 76:77–80, January 1969.

54. Miller JR: Trauma and compensation in gynecology and obstetrics. *Am J Obst Gyn* 26:839–848, December 1933.

55. Baylis SM, et al: Traumatic retroperitoneal hematoma. *Am J Surg* 103:477–480, April 1962.

56. Buchsbaum HJ: How serious is accidental injury during pregnancy? *Med Times* 104:134–137, July 1976.

57. Buchsbaum HJ: Diagnosis and management of abdominal gunshot wounds during pregnancy. *J Trauma* 15:425–430, May 1975.

58. Farzanfar M, Shell JH: Gunshot wounds of the gravid uterus. *J Obst Gyn* 95:877, July 1966.

59. Takki S, et al: Criminal abortion by gunshot. *Annales Chirurgiae et Gynaecologiae Fenniae* 58:122–123, 1969.

60. Nance FC, Cohn I: Surgical judgement in the management of stab wounds of the abdomen. *Ann Surg* 170:569, October 1969.

61. Salomon J, et al: Laceration of the heart in a pregnant woman. *Israel J Med Sci* 6:717–719, November-December 1970.

62. Taylor JW, et al: Thermal injury during pregnancy. *Obst Gyn* 47:434–438, April 1976.

63. Schmitz JT: Pregnant patients with burns. *Am J Obst Gyn* 110:57, May 1971.

64. Toongsuwon S: Postmortem Caesarean section following death by electrocution. *Aust N Zeal J Obst Gyn* 12:265–266, November 1972.

65. Peppler RD, et al: Intrauterine death of a fetus in a mother shocked by an electrical current. *J Louisiana State Med Soc* 124:37–38, February 1972.

66. Rees WD: Pregnant women struck by lightning. *Brit Med J* 1:103–104, January 1965.

67. Gaad RL: The volume of the liquor amnii in normal and abnormal pregnancies. *J Obst Gyn Brit Comm* 73:11–12, February 1966.

68. Rhodes PJ: The volume of liquor amnii in early pregnancy. *J Obst Gyn Brit Comm* 73:23–26, February 1966.

69. London PS: Injury and pregnancy. *Brit J Accident Surg* 6:129–140, November 1974.

70. Alexander E, Davis C: Intra-uterine fracture of the infant's skull. *J Neurosurg* 30:446–454, April 1969.

71. Potter EL: *Pathology of the Fetus and Newborn.* Chicago, Year Book Pub, 1952, p 87.

72. Watson-Jones R: *Fractures and Joint Injuries.* Baltimore, Williams and Wilkins, 1952, p 354.

73. Rothenberger D, et al: Blunt maternal trauma: A review of 103 cases. *J Trauma* 18:173–179, March 1978.

74. Conner E, Curran J: In utero traumatic intraabdominal deceleration injury to the fetus—a case report. *Am J Obst Gyn* 125:567–569, June 1967.

75. Garber EC: Abdominal trauma as a cause of death. *N Carolina Med J* 36:731–732, December 1975.

76. Poulson AM, Gabert HA: Fetal death secondary to nonpenetrating trauma to the gravid uterus. *Am J Obst Gyn* 116:580–582, June 1973.

77. Zivkovic S, et al: Prenatal gunshot perforation of the colon. *J Ped Surg* 11:591–592, August 1976.

78. Gysler R: Intrauterine gunshot wound. *J Ped Surg* 11:589–590, August 1976.

79. Buchsbaum HJ, Caruso PA: Gunshot wound of the pregnant uterus: Case report of fetal injury, deglutition of missile, and survival. *Obst Gyn* 33:673–676, May 1969.

80. Browns R, et al: Thoracoabdominal gunshot wound with survival of a 36-week fetus. *JAMA* 237:2409–2410, May 1977.

81. Barnes AC, Holzman GB: Gynecologic injuries, in Ballinger WF, et al (ed): *The Management of Trauma*. Philadelphia, WB Saunders Co, 1968, pp 409–440.

82. McNebney WK, Smith EI: Penetrating wounds of the gravid uterus. *J Trauma* 12:1024–1028, December 1972.

83. Romney SL, et al: Experimental hemorrhage in late pregnancy. *Am J Obst Gyn* 87:636–649, November 1963.

84. Hakanson EY: Trauma to the female genitalia. *Lancet* 86:287–291, June 1966.

85. Hertig AT: Symposium on problems related to law and surgery: minimal criteria required to prove prima facie case of traumatic abortion or miscarriage; analysis of 1000 spontaneous abortions. *Ann Surg* 117:596–606, April 1943.

86. Nies A: Clinical pharmacology of antihypertensive drugs. *Med Clin N Amer* 61:675–698, May 1977.

87. Steer CM, Petri RH: A comparison of magnesium sulfate and alcohol for the prevention of premature labor. *Am J Obst Gyn* 129:1–4, September 1977.

88. Rothenberger D, et al: Blunt maternal trauma: A review of 103 cases. *J Trauma* 18:173–179, March 1978.

89. Marx GF: Shock in the obstetric patient. *Anesthesiology* 26:423–434, July-August 1965.

90. Romney, et al: Experimental hemorrhage in late pregnancy. *Am J Obst Gyn* 87:636–649, November 1963.

91. Boba A, et al: Effects of vasopressor administration and fluid replacement on fetal bradycardia and hypoxia induced by maternal hemorrhage. *Obst Gyn* 27:408–413, March 1966.

92. Greiss FC: Uterine vascular response to hemorrhage during pregnancy with observations on therapy. *Obst Gyn* 27:549, April 1966.

93. Whitehouse WM, et al: Reduction of radiation hazard in obstetric roentgenography. *Roentgenology* 80:690, 1958.

94. Swartz HM, Reichling BA: The safety of x-ray examination on radioisotope scan. *JAMA* 239:2031–2032, May 1978.

95. Swartz HM, Reichling BA: Hazards of radiation exposure for pregnant women. *JAMA* 239:1907–1908, 1978.

96. Cafferata HT, et al: Intravascular coagulation in the surgical patient. *Am J Surg* 118:281–291, August 1969.

97. Hellman LM, Pritchard JA: Maternal physiology in pregnancy, in *William's Obstetrics*. New York, Appleton-Century-Crofts, 1971, p 236.

98. Phillips LL, et al: Hemorrhage due to fibrinolysis in abruptio placentae. *Am J Obst Gyn* 84:1447–1456, December 1962.

99. Olcott C, et al: Amniotic fluid embolism and disseminated intravascular coagulation after blunt abdominal trauma. *J Trauma* 13:737–740, August 1973.

100. String T, et al: Massive trauma: Effect of intravascular coagulation on prognosis. *Arch Surg* 102:406–411, April 1971.

101. Pacey J, et al: Peritoneal tap and lavage in patients with blunt abdominal trauma: Their contribution to surgical decisions. *Canad Med Ass J* 105:365–370, August 1971.

102. Buchsbaum HJ: Accidental injury complicating pregnancy. *Am J Obst Gyn* 102:752–769, November 1968.

103. Rothenberger DA, et al: Diagnostic peritoneal lavage for blunt trauma in pregnant women. *Am J Obst Gyn* 129:479–481, November 1977.

104. Perry JF: A five-year survey of 152 acute abdominal injuries. *J Trauma* 5:53–61, January 1965.

The Management of Mass Casualty Disasters

Frank J. Baker, II, M.D.
Associate Professor and Director
Department of Emergency Medicine
The University of Chicago Hospitals and
*   Clinics*
Chicago, Illinois

THE ABILITY OF health care professionals to manage mass casualty disasters has improved dramatically with the development of emergency medical services systems. Management principles have evolved from the application of tested military concepts to civilian practice. Development of efficient communications, on-site response by medical personnel, rapid field triage and stabilization and ambulance dispatch are components of a planned process to manage mass casualties most efficiently.

The major difficulty in managing mass casualty disasters is limited resources. This problem is not, however, limited to the medical community, but includes all public agencies, such as police and fire departments, as well as charitable organizations, such as the American Red Cross and the Salvation Army. During a disaster, the number of victims with acute medical problems frequently exceeds the medical community's resources to deal with them.

150 The rational approach is to provide maximum benefit to the greatest number of victims while deploying limited resources. Only by careful planning can such an objective be realized.

The planning process has been discussed sufficiently in the literature.[1-8] Suffice it to say that in the planning process the agency responsible for developing a mass casualty disaster plan and the agency with overall operational responsibility at the disaster site must be identified. All agencies involved in the actual management of a disaster must be included in an active program. The military should always be included since it may assume overall operational authority in a major disaster.[9] The disaster program should be continually tested, critiqued and redesigned, so that the operational plan will always build on demonstrated strengths. Furthermore, operational flexibility is necessary if the plan is to be workable.[6,7,10-13]

In general, the incidence of technological disasters has increased in recent times. There obviously were no airplane crashes prior to the age of flight, and no bus accidents prior to the invention of the internal combustion engine. As society becomes more sophisticated and more urbanized, and as our technology becomes more complex, the possibilities for major disruption to that technology increase. As our society moves toward mass transportation, mass housing and mass gatherings, the threat of disaster increases. The incidence of natural disasters will not decrease significantly in the foreseeable future, and thus the net incidence of disasters with attendant large numbers of casualties will increase.

COMMUNICATIONS

Communication is a universal problem in any disaster.[1,14-16] The bystander who first observes the occurrence may be unable to report it immediately because of such mundane problems as lack of change for a pay telephone or not knowing which agency to notify. These seemingly trivial problems are real and could be of critical import, since valuable minutes in the immediate postdisaster period that might allow public safety agencies to limit the scope of the disaster may be lost. This can best be remedied by the institution of a 911 emergency telephone system, which is being established with increasing frequency in the United States.

Notification of public safety agencies, such as police and fire departments, immediately mobilizes manpower and equipment, since these agencies usually have well-designed, written protocols governing their response to specific situations. A major and almost universal problem has been the general inability of police and fire departments to provide timely notification of a disaster to hospitals. This is actually to be expected, since police and fire departments cannot justify the routine staffing of communications facilities the size required to maintain efficient communications during a disaster. In addition, their primary role is the management of the public safety aspects of any disaster and therefore notification of hospitals and medical personnel assumes a temporary, secondary importance.

The hospitals must be promptly notified so that timely decisions can be made regarding the mobilization of medical teams from hospitals.

A decision to send hospital-based medical teams to the disaster site must be made on the scene by medical professionals. When such decisions are made by public safety personnel without medical training, the result is usually a "load-and-go" approach ignoring the modern concepts of field triage and stabilization, and resulting in inadequate patient care.[17] Hospitals require a lead time to organize and transport the medical teams and to prepare their facilities to receive inordinate numbers of patients.

To notify hospitals of a disaster, Chicago uses a unique system based on the Mobile Intensive Care Unit (MICU) system, which employs advanced life-support vehicles staffed by paramedics. The city is divided into three regions, each with its own resource hospital, which is the only institution in that area communicating over the airwaves to the ambulances. The resource hospital is connected to participating hospitals in the region through a system of dedicated telephone lines. Daily, these dedicated lines relay information about patients to hospitals receiving patients via the MICU system.

The Chicago Fire Department (CFD), which operates and staffs the MICU vehicles in conjunction with the participating hospitals, no longer notifies every hospital receiving patients of a disaster, but instead alerts only the MICU resource hospital for the region in which the disaster occurs. This significantly decreases the communications traffic generated at CFD and allows for the notification of the resource hospital in the first minutes of a disaster. The resource hospital, using the MICU dedicated telephone lines, collates information from the receiving hospitals on the status of the emergency department, intensive care section and blood banks. Using this information and communications with the disaster site, including the number and type of injuries, the resource hospital notifies the participating hospitals to send medical teams to the site, receive disaster victims or remain on standby alert. These critical determinants of patient distribution are also relayed to the ambulance dispatch site. This system has decreased average hospital notification time from 20 minutes to less than five minutes and permits rational dispatch of ambulances to the most appropriate hospitals. This has been documented during a number of actual disasters.[18]

ON-SITE MEDICAL PERSONNEL

Prior to the development of the paramedic MICU systems, on-site medical personnel were usually hospital-based medical teams. The delay in their response, coupled with the sometimes prolonged evacuation procedure and the all-too-frequent "load-and-go" operation, is associated with increased morbidity and mortality in patients with insecure airways, hypovolemic shock and unstable fractures. Despite the advent of prehospital MICU systems, hospital-based teams are a necessity in disasters, since many mass casualty incidents involve prolonged evacuation. In addition, the sheer number of casualties may overwhelm paramedic systems alone. Hospital medical staff should be trained in triage and field stabilization, and should be transported to the disaster site with appropriate medical equipment, protective gear and identification.[19,20] A unique solution has been devised in Chicago by the adop-

152 tion of a green hard hat marked "Emergency Medical Team" as the official identification permitting access to the disaster site. The advantage of this identification is that it is protective and immediately visible, facilitating ready field identification of medical teams at the disaster site, even though the geographical area of the site may be quite large.

RAPID FIELD TRIAGE

The institution of MICU systems in many cities has replaced medically untrained fire and police personnel with trained medical personnel as the first help at the disaster site. Prior to this development, it was nearly impossible to convince public safety agencies of the advantages of rapid field triage and stabilization. In many respects, the rapid transportation philosophy evolved because in the past these individuals had little medical training. The result, of course, was the deadly "load-and-go" operation that has been witnessed at many disasters. Field triage and stabilization has been credited with reducing mortality in the Moorgate Tube train disaster in London in 1975 and the Loop "L" train wreck in Chicago in 1977.[2,16,21]

Rapid field triage, coupled with stabilization by paramedics must be directed from a Medical Command Post (MCP) at the disaster site. All paramedics and hospital-based medical teams must report to the MCP before going into the actual disaster site. The MCP coordinates medical operations, establishes triage, decides on the appropriateness and location of field hospitals and the site and operation of the ambulance dispatch area. Personnel at the MCP are also responsible for the allocation of material resources, and must have a direct communications link with the MICU resource hospital, which coordinates the hospital-based aspects of these operations.

The first priority is to obtain an overview of the severity of the disaster and the resources available. Only then can clinical triage begin. Rapid field triage should be performed by the first medical personnel on the scene, and the initial triage process should follow an algorithm (see Figure 1) consisting of initial assessment of breathing and consciousness. Apneic patients should be presumed dead and labeled as such. Patients with labored breathing, or who are unconscious, should have immediate airway stabilization. Significant numbers of mass casualty victims die of traumatic asphyxia.[16] While the patient with respiratory distress may respond to simple airway maneuvers, it is doubtful that a patient with apnea as a result of trauma will respond to these maneuvers. After airway stabilization, all survivors should have a quick visual assessment, aimed at categorizing them as critical, urgent or ambulatory wounded. Specific treatment rendered at this point should be limited to direct compression or dressing of potentially exsanguinating hemorrhages and dressing of sucking chest wounds. Triage personnel should not spend an inordinate amount of time on any single patient before determination of the priorities of care for all of the patients at the disaster site. Medical teams can later return to the most critical patients and begin field stabilization.

A four-color, coded triage system and

FIGURE 1.   INITIAL TRIAGE PROCESS

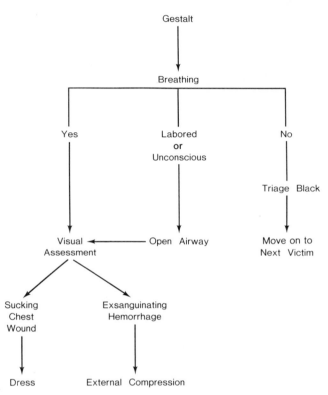

standard triage tag should be used, since it is the easiest method to use and remember. Utilization of a standard disaster tag facilitates rapid field triage, since most hospital-based medical teams responding to a disaster in general are not intimately familiar with details of the local disaster plan.[22] Chicago has adopted the triage tag designed by the *Journal of Civil Defense* located in Starke, Florida. (See Figure 2.) This tag is ideal in that it allows for identification of the patient, as well as the listing of critical information such as the patient's injuries and the medications received. In addition, it is clearly symbol-

and color-coded and extremely easy to use. Category 0 (or black) indicates an expired victim. Category 1 (or red) is used for the critical patient whose survival is dependent on immediate stabilization of a life threat. Category 2 (or yellow) indicates an urgently or seriously injured patient who requires some medical stabilization in the field prior to transportation, but whose life is not immediately threatened. Category 3 (or green) is applied to the ambulatory or walking wounded patient who does not require any medical attention at the disaster site prior to transporation to a hospital.

154 **FIGURE 2. MEDICAL EMERGENCY TRIAGE TAG (METTAG)**

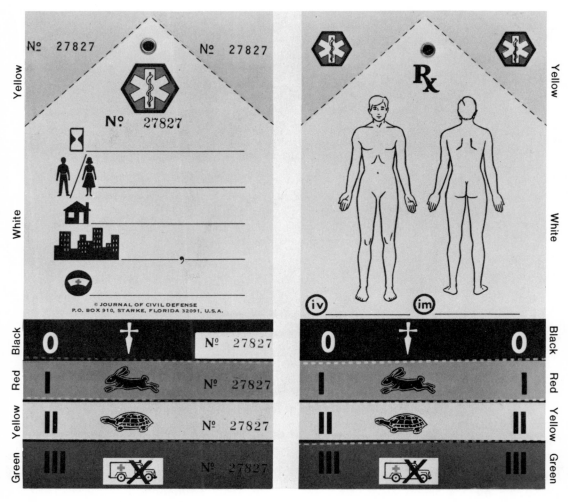

With this particular tag, one simply detaches the inappropriate colors and leaves the appropriate classification color at the bottom of the tag. This triage system assumes that patients will not be retriaged on the field from a more to a less serious category.
Source: *Journal of Civil Defense,* Starke, Florida.

The use of the four-color triage system depends on the flexibility and judgment of on-site medical personnel in assessing the availability of medical resources and making independent decisions categoriz-

ing those near death. If on-site resources to care for the critically injured prior to transportation are inadequate, the 100% burn patient, for example, is categorized as expired and receives no treatment. On the other hand, this same patient, if resources permit, may be categorized as a critical patient and receives analgesic therapy in a humanitarian effort to relieve pain. Providing the maximum care for the greatest number of patients, aimed at maximum survival, must always be kept in mind. The operational plan must allow medical personnel the flexibility to make these judgments.

FIELD STABILIZATION

After assessment and categorization, medical personnel should move into the next phase of the disaster plan, stabilization prior to transport. The medical aspect consists of stabilizing airway and breathing, and stopping hemorrhage. If adequate rapid field triage has been performed, the most important aspect of stabilization is the treatment of hypovolemic shock with fluid resuscitation. This procedure along with stabilizing fractures is, in many instances, the limit of what can be done in the field for the patient.

Flexibility, again, remains the key since the size of the disaster and the location and the availability of resources will determine whether the patients should be stabilized where they lie in the field or whether field hospitals should be established. (See Figure 3.) It is conceivable that in a major disaster at a remote locale, with large numbers of victims and few medical facilities nearby, the patients may remain for up to 24 hours in field hospitals prior to transport to a hospital for more definitive care. In this situation, the stabilization phase may involve surgical procedures, sophisticated ventilatory manage-

FIGURE 3. TRIAGE PROCEDURE FOR DISASTER VICTIMS

155

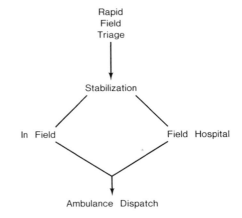

ment and continued treatment of shock. This would, however, be the exception rather than the rule; in most circumstances, particularly in metropolitan areas, stabilization of victims in the field will be done at the disaster site itself, rather than in a field hospital set up at the periphery of the disaster site.

AMBULANCE DISPATCH AND TRANSPORT

In general, transportation to the hospital has not been handled well by public safety personnel, again, because of rapid "load-and-go" techniques which preclude rational patient distribution. The emphasis on speed and sirens and the resulting increase in the number of motor vehicle accidents involving ambulances have led to higher morbidity and mortality rates for patients as well as emergency medical service personnel. The priority for removing patients from the site is as follows:

156 critical patients (red) first; followed by the urgent patients (yellow); next the walking wounded (green); and finally the expired patients (black). However, the priority of removal should take into account the degree of stabilization that has occurred on site and the ability of emergency medical service personnel to care for the patients before and during transport. In addition, the ability of hospitals to care for the patients they will receive must be a prime factor in determining the numbers, triage categories and destinations of the patients.

These decisions should be made at ambulance dispatch by an individual with medical expertise in conjunction with a public safety officer who is knowledgeable about ambulance dispatch. Only in this way can ambulance dispatch proceed with a methodical, rational distribution of patients and avoid sending patients to institutions with limited resources that cannot provide optimal care for the victims. Ambulance dispatch must take into account information from the resource hospital about the capabilities of its receiving institutions to care for the various types of patients. This assessment of resources should be a continuing process during the entire operation.

Patients arriving at individual institutions will need retriage since some unfortunately will have deteriorated. It is usually not necessary or possible to perform retriage in the field. When retriage is performed, whatever its location, it is extremely hazardous to place a patient into a less serious category. For example, a patient categorized as yellow in the field because of a femoral fracture is much more likely to deteriorate to category red than improve to category green. Mistakenly classifying injuries into a more serious class will rarely result in overtreatment, whereas erroneous retriage into a less severe category may result in not treating a life-threatening problem.

After the disaster site has been cleared of all victims, hospitals should be notified that no more victims will be transported. Interhospital disaster communications should remain operational to assist in patient transfer to specialty units and hospitals, and in the possible transfer of necessary drugs and supplies from one institution to another. In the immediate postdisaster phase the medical community must be prepared to deal with the psychological and psychiatric problems which are known to occur in both victims and health care professionals.[23]

There is little doubt that mistakes will always be made in the management of mass casualty disasters due to the variability of circumstances. Maximum flexibility of a plan is necessary to insure efficient operation. Therefore, after the disaster, all the agencies involved should conduct a private, direct and forthright critique of the management of the disaster. The goal of the critique should be correcting weaknesses and building strengths. Proposed changes should be tested in regular disaster drills. Only through planning, preparation, practice and continual revision can the medical community, in conjunction with public safety officials, hope to provide the greatest help to victims of a mass casualty disaster.

SUMMARY

Common problems in the management of mass casualties include communication, response by hospital-based personnel, triage, field stabilization and patient distri-bution through an on-site ambulance dispatch area. Planning, coupled with maximum flexibility and routine practice, all insure maximum patient benefit when a mass casualty situation arises.

REFERENCES

1. Jelenko C, et al: *Emergency Medical Services—An Overview.* Bowie, Maryland, Robert J Brady Co, 1976, pp 213–217, 265–279.
2. King EG: The moorgate disaster: lessons for the internist. *Ann Intern Med*, 84:333–334, 1975.
3. Schwartz GR, et al: *The Principles and Practice of Emergency Medicine.* Philadelphia, WB Saunders Co, 1978, pp 1422–1427.
4. Gibson G: *Emergency Medical Services in the Chicago Area.* Chicago, Center of Health Administration Studies, University of Chicago Press, 1970, p 161.
5. Bohn GA, Richie CG: Learning by simulation: the validation of disaster simulation: medical scheme planning. *J Kansas Med Soc*, 1:418–425, November 1970.
6. Holloway RM: Medical disaster planning: urban areas. *New York J Med*, 71:591–595, 692–694, March 1971.
7. Conrad MB, Klippel AP: Disaster planning in a metropolitan area. *Bulletin Amer Coll Surg* 57:19–22, May 1972.
8. Hollis TL, Sapp BW: The hospital as an emergency center. *JAHA* 46:38–41, May 1972.
9. Stalcup SA, Oscherwitz M, Cohen MS, et al: Planning for a pediatric disaster—experience gained from caring for 1600 Vietnamese orphans. *N Engl J Med*, 293(14):691–695, 1975.
10. Rutherford WH: Experience in the accident and emergency department of the Royal Victoria Hospital with patients from civil disturbances in Belfast 1964–1972, with a review of disasters in the United Kingdom 1951–1971. *Injury* 4:189–199, 1973.
11. Hart RJ, Lee JO, Boyles DJ, et al: The summerland disaster. *Brit Med J* 1:256–259, 1975.
12. Hays MB, Stefanki JX, Cheu DB: Planning an airport disaster drill. *Space Environ Med* 47(5):56–60, 1976.
13. Clark CD: The need for mock major accidents. *Resuscitation* 4(4):283–284, 1975.
14. Ballinger W: *The Management of Trauma* ed 2. Philadelphia, WB Saunders Co, 1973, p 761.
15. Owens JC: Emergency health services require efficient communications system. *JAHA* 42:71–72, June 1969.
16. Members of the Medical Staff of Three London Hospitals: Moorgate tube train disaster. *Brit Med J* 3:727–731, 1975.
17. Minutes: Critique of the Horween Leather Factory disaster. Papers of the Emergency Medical Services Commission of the Metropolitan Chicago Disaster Preparedness Committee, Chicago, Chicago Hospital Council, 1978.
18. Minutes: Critique of the Wincrest Nursing Home fire. Papers of the Emergency Medical Services Commission of the Metropolitan Chicago Disaster Preparedness Committee, Chicago, Chicago Hospital Council, 1976.
19. Strickler A: The case of disaster site medical teams. *Dimens Health Serv* 53(2):30–32, February 1976.
20. Savage BE: Disaster planning: protective clothing for medical teams. *Injury* 7(4):286–287, May 1976.
21. Minutes: Critique of the Chicago Transit Authority Loop elevated train crash. Papers of the Emergency Medical Services Commission of the Metropolitan Chicago Disaster Preparedness Committee, Chicago, Chicago Hospital Council, 1978.
22. Prepared for a disaster, editorial. *Brit Med J*, 3:723, September 1975.
23. Parad H, Resnik H, Parad L (eds): *Emergency and Disaster Management: A Mental Health Sourcebook.* Bowie, Maryland, Charles Press Publisher, 1976, pp 209–392.

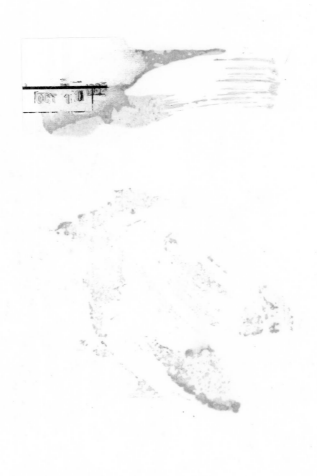